Stumbling In Flats

A funny old life with MS...

Barbara A. Stensland

Barbara A Stensland

Justifiedtext.co.uk   ISBN 978-0-9926088-6-6

@DebbieBarlow5 - Love your blog I must say!! It's just like reading my own life!! X

@John127Joyce - Great blog yet again. You hit the nail on the head every time x

@jojochester - Love your blogs, I have a little cheer when I see you have written a new one!! Xx

@helenahorne - Am recently diagnosed and have only just discovered your blog. Absolutely love it. Helps loads.

@TheMSKittylady - Brilliant as always – you're a fab writer Xx

@Soupdragon1965 - Your blogs make me laugh out loud, and brighten up the bad days/bad moments.

@jennywilsonbest - Once again great blog. You make me feel less alone with my MS.

@catdoran - Read your blog from start to finish last night. Brilliantly written, was nodding my head in agreement at so much.

@carlysoffe86 - LOVE your blog. I can relate to so much. It really makes a difference to my day.

@shiremoorpotter - An outstanding form of words: 'divorced single parent, with Teenager, cat, MS and compost heap'.

@flookoco- You have a great blog! My other half has MS and your blog is a great support.

@RobynMeme - I like waking up to one of your inspiring blogs.

@phillipses - I think you're an amazing person and you've been such a support to me over the past 9 months since my dx. You're invaluable.

@annthepoet - I always enjoy your writing and feel a connection. You're great at saying it how it is ☺ X

@ellexbee - I can relate to everything you write, love your blogs.

@AndreaLisher - Just read your blog for the first time, it's brilliant ☺

@verity_leah - Just wanted to say that I really love your blog. Beautifully written.

@cab6287 - Your blogs are brilliant, they make me smile and I relate to them!! Love the writing style!

@shandymitford - Recently diagnosed with MS and came across your blog. Thank you!! X

@MsAmandaEllen - I don't say it enough, but I love your blog!

@suzyp5 - Please stop writing what I think but far more eloquently than I ever could!

@Stevekitzinger - Thank you so much for what you have written, my feelings exactly, but I couldn't find the words.

Acknowledgements

With huge thanks to:

My mum, Barbara Stensland-Sloane, for always being there for me.

My auntie, Elizabeth Morrison, for keeping it real.

My long-suffering friend and boss, Tony Smith.

Caroline Tidy, who makes the best cakes ever.

Janis H. Winehouse, for her kind words and encouragement.

Everyone in the MS team at the University Hospital of Wales, Cardiff - for being brilliant and giving the best care possible: my neurologist, Dr T. Pickersgill and all the MS nurses - Jacki Smee, Gail Clayton, Rhiannon Jones, Sian Locke and Lynn Kelly Jones.

Dr Eleanor Davies - my wonderful GP.

The MS Society, UK, MS Trust, Shift-ms – between them, these organisations are an incredible source of information, support and research.

Paul Eustice, publisher extraordinaire, who has expertly guided me through the whole process.

Everyone who read my blog and all those who posted comments **– this book would not be here without you!**

For Christopher, The Teenager

In memory of my dad, John Andreas Stensland
1943 - 1978
Who never had the same MS treatment options as I have had.
I love and miss you and always will.

Foreword, by Janis H. Winehouse

Being a lady of a certain age (60) I had no idea what a blog is! My research led me down several avenues, some quite dubious, but eventually the concept dawned on me.

Just after the birth of my son Alex 35 years ago, I started to get strange sensations. I felt tired, my energy levels dropped and I was at a loss as to what was going on. Like most people, my GP was a logical person to visit, then followed tests at the hospital all of which proved inconclusive and although MS was suggested it was quickly forgotten about!

Life continued with the birth of Amy and my resources were books, which offered little and I never knew anyone in a similar situation.

2003 was the turning point for me. I had been slowing down quite a bit but I picked up a virus while I was in Italy and I had revenge on Vesuvius when I threw up on it! Back in England tests finally showed I had secondary progressive MS. It seems I missed the relapsing and remitting part, but had I been computer savvy and found a blog I would have realised much earlier what was wrong and that there are thousands of us out there, I was not alone.

The value of the Stumbling in Flats blog, and indeed all social media, is it opens so many avenues of support and understanding, not only to the sufferer but to the family, the friends, the social workers and all those carers who come into our lives, so that they will understand what it's like to walk through treacle, to stumble in the street, to fall asleep at the drop of a hat and all the other indignities which we may or may not go through. We can do anything our bodies will let us we try to lead normal lives. We have MS.

JHW 2015

Introduction - From Running in Heels to Stumbling in Flats

The day before MS crashed into my life, things were on the up.

I had a rewarding job, which would hopefully lay the foundation for a second degree in Health and Social Care, which could ultimately lead to an MA in Social Work, which would get me back on my somewhat fractured career ladder after working part-time and taking on full responsibility for my son's childcare.

So, life was great. Until the morning I woke up unable to string a sentence together. My speech was shot to pieces, my balance similarly so. Something was very, very wrong.

It took just one day to turn my world on its head. A bewildering array of medical procedures followed – a lumbar puncture, scans, endless blood tests and exercises where I walked corridors with someone following me with a round thing on a stick and drink-driving tests where I had to touch my neurologist's nose with my finger and walk in a straight line (not at the same time, thankfully, although his aftershave was strangely intoxicating).

I was sent away with a handful of MS leaflets and a Relapse Hotline Number. But I didn't have MS? Yet. The clue is in the diagnosis, 'multiple'. I had to wait for another relapse and it didn't take long.

I was 'lucky' – my relapses popped up so frequently I was eligible for Campath (Alemtuzumab) but it wasn't enough to save me from being sacked from a job I loved, just for having MS.

Yes, I fought back. And yup, I struggled through baffling brain fog to finish the degree. I thought at one point I had a new job (two interviews!) but alas, they mothballed the project due to the recession. Anyway, I threw my towel in and signed up for a Master's in Creative Writing instead and started working for my friend's company. And so a different future began.

I also started a blog to share my frustrations, fears and feelings with others and quickly discovered a wonderful online community. After over two years of publishing random thoughts about life with MS, I was persuaded to compile a selection together into a book.

And here it is …

24th September 2012

In The Beginning, There Was Cake …

Like so many things in my life, MS began with cake.

Leaving a friend's house after enjoying a slice (okay, two slices) of delicious cake. I turned to say, 'thanks for the cake!' but it came out as 'thanks, Kate'. Odd. I tried again. Same thing.

I went home perplexed. The Teenager was away for the weekend and over the course of the next two days my speech deteriorated, I was exhausted and my balance was shot. I knew something was seriously wrong.

I eventually ended up in hospital, talking gibberish. The clues were all there; the overwhelming tiredness over the previous six months, the dodgy walking, the simplest tasks taking forever. Throw in a parent who'd had MS and I guessed the rest.

I assumed I would be diagnosed there and then (ha!) but that was just the beginning. Until I had a further relapse, I was in Limboland with no idea how long I would stay there. It took a year to hear the dreaded words, 'highly active/rapidly evolving relapsing remitting MS'.

That year was probably the worst of my life. The lumbar puncture was vile, the MRIs terrifying and I lost

3

count of how many blood tests I had. I lay awake at night, rigid with fear, worrying about the future.

A lot of people say the day they are finally diagnosed is both the best and worst day of their lives. I agree. After all the waiting, the anxiety, the fears, it was a relief to finally have some answers. But it doesn't make it any easier.

My main priority was to keep life going on as normal as possible for The Teenager. I would sleep in the afternoons, setting my alarm so I was awake just before he got home from school, duvet tucked away behind the sofa. I hid my anxiety. I became best friends with the pizza delivery man.

Those were dark, dark days. The worst of them are behind me now and an uncertain future still lies ahead, but isn't that true for everyone?

And as for cake, well, it certainly hasn't put me off...

26th September 2012

Introducing The Teenager

Teenagers, eh? Don't you just love 'em? To be fair, I've got a pretty decent model. So far.

Anyway, it was hard enough beginning to come to terms with *me* having MS, far less breaking it to him. He knew there was something wrong, he just wasn't sure what. He realised I was tired, a bit snappier than usual and I was traipsing back and forward to the hospital, the doctor's, etc.

I was very organised. I had already ordered a kid's guide to MS, full of reassuring pictures in primary colours and simple text. So, we had to have The Conversation. The scene was set. I had cooked his favourite dinner, presented him with dessert (normally only on a Sunday), and managed to pin him to the sofa long enough to have a heart-to-heart. It went something like this:

Me: Um, you know, yes. Well, it's like this. See?

Him: Uh, no?

Me: Well, you know all those appointments I've been having? It seems I have something called multiple sclerosis. Nothing to worry about. Oh, and here's a little guide for you to have a read of. In your own time, you know? Now, is there anything you want to ask me?

Him: D'uh. Like, I know? Like, I'm on all the forums. I can even pronounce it. I know all about it. Can I go now?

Me: I really think we should talk about this.

Him: Ok. Are you going to die?

Me: Not from MS, no.

Him: Will you be in a wheelchair?

Me: Not for a really long while, if at all.

Him: (jumps up) Cool. See ya!

And there you have it; how *not* to have an awkward conversation with The Teenager.

28th September 2012

Friday At Last

I only work a couple of days a week, having dropped some hours (thanks, MS!) but I still get out-of-proportion excited whenever Friday rolls around.

Only one problem with that: my expectations way exceed reality. I sit there in work, idly scrolling through events listings, checking out the live music pages, the theatre, the cinema, new restaurant openings and all the rest of it.

In my mind, I'm dressed up like a goddess on steroids and even have some fabulously high heels on. My hair is swishy, my make-up is flawless and I have a zinging, Friday-night energy. I picture myself surrounded by glossy, admiring friends, casually toasting each other in some brand-new bar, attracting envious yet welcoming stares from handsome men.

I will be on top form, wowing my friends with incredible stories gleaned over my busy week and perhaps impressing them by throwing a delicately-spiced wasabi nut in the air and catching it effortlessly in my mouth. Or I will be hanging out at the more alternative arts place, with my black polo neck and smart, slightly-distressed jeans on, accessorised with chunky, hand-made beads from a women's collective in The Gambia. With my beret at a jaunty angle, I will toss out witty remarks, only pausing to applaud the experimental jazz band playing in the corner.

We will drink Belgian-brewed gooseberry cider and dip artisan bread in olive oil flavoured with crushed Chilean peppers.

Which one do I choose?

Well, neither. At the end of the week I'm shattered, my sofa has been calling me and I just about have enough energy to peel the lid from a microwave meal.

So, the reality? Me, in pyjamas, face-pack on, watching other people have fabulous nights out on telly.

30th September 2012

I Kid You Not

MS has made me more adventurous and given me a desire to 'try new things'. I'm not sure why, perhaps a case of, what have I got to lose? I have an ongoing list of new things to try, more often added to than attempted. Yesterday, I set out to change this.

Every weekend I buy a small child's height of newspapers and every weekend I read the recipe pages, scanning through the ingredients, the cooking methods, the time taken, think, 'hmm, that sounds nice' and quickly turn the page, berating myself for not exposing The Teenager to more exotic food.

But yesterday, I promised myself that I would try out the first recipe I came across. Perhaps I should have read The Mail on Saturday first (Jamie's 15 minute meals - desserts this week, darn it), but I picked up The Guardian as I always turn to the 'Blind Date' article - living vicariously.

The divine Hugh Fearnley-Whittingstall is leaning casually against his Aga, pots hanging from a driftwood rack behind him. He asks, 'why don't we eat more goat?'

Oh. Um, because the local Co-op doesn't stock it?

But in the spirit of adventure, I read on. Perhaps Waitrose have it. Or that obscure butcher I always mean to visit (another tick on 'try new things' list). First ingredient is hay. This is not going well.

Helpfully though, Hugh suggests that if I don't know a farmer, I can always buy small packs of it from a pet shop. Ok, quick visit to Pets At Home too, then.

So, assuming I have my goat and my hay, the next thing I have to do is to soak the hay in a bucket, then drain. I don't have a bucket, long story. Quick trip to the hardware store too then, Hugh? Nope.

Take the goat, the hay and the bucket off my shopping list, scribble down chops, potatoes and veg. Maybe try again next week, but for now, reading the recipe was adventurous enough.

1st October 2012

An Electric Feeling

One of the many symptoms of MS I had yet to
experience properly has struck with full force. Those
electric shock sensations, also known as l'Hermittes sign,
had up until now only bothered me fleetingly, lasting no
more than a couple of seconds each time.

I was helping a friend strip wallpaper over the weekend
(I know, the excitement), when they started up. A bit like
labour pains, there was some time between each to start
with, but they slowly increased until it was an almost
continuous pain.

I won't bore you with the details, but the sensation was
so strange and so bizarrely painful, I laid down my tools,
got in the car and slowly drove home, a journey made
more difficult as I couldn't move my head and a tractor
had broken down in the middle of the road.

And there's the nub. Just when you think you have MS
under control, it decides to stick a hand in its big bag of
symptoms and chuck another one at you.

It's amazing what you can come to regard as normal -
the tiredness, the dodgy walking, the balance problems, the
twitching, the numb hands, the overwhelming desire to
stuff my face with chocolate - and you adjust your life
accordingly.

Everything is as good as it can be, until something like this knocks you back to square one again. I've been wondering though, how did MS'ers describe the pain before electricity was invented?

3rd October 2012

Job Centre Blues

After burrowing around in the murky depths of disability and work legislation, I have been assigned a Disability Employment Advisor and on Monday I went to visit her at the local Job Centre.

To cut a very long, sorry saga short, I have been bullied quite viciously at work ever since my diagnosis of multiple sclerosis and I need to find a new job. Pronto. Can you *believe* this is still happening in 2012?

Anyway, I'm told to bring my CV and turn up at 11.20 sharp. I arrive early and am met by two doormen. Bouncers? Honestly, they stand there in dark suits, look me up and down with raised eyebrows and I'm half expecting them to say 'sorry love, you can't come in here looking like that'.

I'm directed into a vast, bland, utterly depressing room with splashes of green logo and dotted with a bewildering array of prams, shopping bags and people slumped on the sofas. Other people are hunched over large 'job generating machines', pressing and clicking buttons like they're playing one-armed bandits in a pub.

I pick my way through the crowd, perch on the edge of a threadbare sofa and wait. And wait. The staff call people up to desks, looking bored out their skulls (well, they already have jobs) and still I wait, my CV wilting in my sweaty hand.

Finally, I'm called. We run through the ways MS can get in the way of working, my skills, my career aspirations and which hours I can work. My advisor then turns the computer screen round so I can see it. Two possible jobs. Cleaning and daytime pizza delivery. Huh?

She tells me I'm over-qualified for most of the jobs they have, but due to my reduced working hours, childcare issues and disability, that's all they can offer.

I thank her, walk unsteadily to the door with as much dignity as I can and leave it all behind. On second thoughts, I go back, slip past the bouncers and yank a 'How Did We Do?' form from the front desk. On it I write Abandon Hope All Ye Who Enter Here, shove it in the box and go.

4th October 2012

It's All Me, Me, Me

Having MS, just how hard is it to show sympathy to people who are a little under the weather but who make a lot of noise about it?

Has MS made me less compassionate, and do I somehow think no one else has the right to moan to me about their own troubles?

I only ask as two friends and The Teenager have recently been struck down with bad colds. All three are male, so naturally 'man flu' has been mooted as a possibility but, to be fair, they do seem very poorly and I am trying to be sympathetic, listen attentively and give helpful suggestions. I care about these people and hate to see them ill.

But a teeny-tiny-little part of me thinks it's a bit like expecting a poor person to empathise with a rich guy when his Porsche is in the garage for repairs.

Sure, it's an inconvenience, but it's temporary and normal service will resume soon enough. I want to say, 'Ill? *You're* ill? You *want* to see what ill is?'

How awful is that? What sort of person am I to even think that? I have bored my friends to tears over the last year, constantly dissecting symptoms to the nth degree, analysing lesions and spilling out my fears for the future. They have sat with me through a merry-go-round of appointments, held my hand during MRI's and kept my glass of wine topped up.

So I feel very small-minded to begrudge them that little bit of extra attention and help when they need it. I have offered to drive 18 miles through the rain to bring supplies to one friend and have tucked The Teenager up in bed with a book and hot Lemsip. This is one battle the MS Monster won't win. MS may be for life, but so are friends and family.

5th October 2012

Chocolate Dreams

Chocolate haunts me. Last night a giant Jaffa Cake chased me down the road. When I woke up, I could almost taste it. I adore chocolate and it worships me in return. So much so that it hangs around my thighs, stubbornly clinging on for dear life.

I know we need to go our separate ways, but it's a really comforting friend to have around. Always available, cheap and comes in endless varieties so you never get bored.

MS has given me a great excuse - when the worst has already happened, who cares if you treat yourself now and again? So many other things seem more important than whether I'm knocking back the chocolate buttons by the bucket-load.

Just had an excruciating lumbar puncture? Have a family-sized Galaxy bar. Fallen flat on your face in a packed restaurant? Order a profiterole surprise to share then grab both forks.

In a desperate bid to curb my cravings, I came up with a cunning plan. Advent calendars are on sale now. What if I were to buy one and *only* pop open two windows a day? Plus, I'll get some early Christmassy vibes going.

I reached Christmas Eve that same night and put the pillaged calendar out for recycling.

Ok, Plan B. Eat *no* chocolate all week, then have a blow-out on Friday. I was cured! I ate so much of the stuff, I vowed never to eat it again, until I woke up on Saturday and noticed there were still a few Maltesers left in the packet...

6th October 2012

Interview Nerves

Is it just me or are job interviews like blind dates?

You need to make a dazzling impression in 3 seconds flat, you spend ages on your outfit and you practice your witty laugh and come-back comments in the mirror.

I had an interview yesterday and I always reckon Friday interviews are a good bet - everyone's looking forward to the weekend and we can just kick back and chill. Wouldn't you know though, it was a job I applied for and promptly forgot about as I was only asked to submit my CV and a covering email. Yet I can spend hours and hours on carefully-crafted, 10-page long personal statements and not hear a peep.

Anyway, I took an inordinate amount of time selecting a suitable outfit, painstakingly applied make-up so that it looked like I wasn't wearing any, teased my unruly hair into bouncy waves and applied perfume liberally.

I read up on the company, memorised facts and wrote a few tiny crib notes on my wrist, carefully hidden under my watch. Unfortunately, as this whole process took over two hours, I downed gallons of coffee to steady my nerves.

By the time I left the house, every nerve was buzzing, but, hey, I was on form, I was flying.

At the reception desk, a jaded receptionist slapped a very large ID sticker on my coat and commanded me to sit and wait until I was 'collected'.

I was then lead to *the* most open-plan office ever designed where the workers were handing round birthday cake, casting sympathetic little glances in my direction, as I huddled in the tiny corner sitting-area. Finally I was called in to The Panel and an hour (an hour!) later, I was led back to the lift, unpeeled from my sticker and sent on my way.

I won't be cracking open the Champagne just yet, but I think I have a good chance. If I'm successful I get called back for a second, then a third interview, gulp. Wish me luck and watch this space...

7th October 2012

Just Chop It All Off...

In my continuing quest to 'try new things', I decided to chop most of my hair off yesterday. I usually steer clear of hair salons as much as possible because:

- I'm a whole generation older than most of the clients, grrr

- I'm not ready for a bubble perm and tint just yet

- I never, ever get the cut I ask for

Yet I was feeling strangely optimistic and full of hope as I tried a new hairdresser.

I was given a look book, a strong coffee and the latest copy of Vogue. A child glided over and picked up my locks, tutted, exchanged glances with the child next to her and just about managed not to roll her eyes. I know, I know, I've let my whole hair-care regime lapse into grunge since being diagnosed with MS. It's not been that high up on my list of priorities, but that's all about to change.

The child, who turned out to be a mother-of-two, asked me what look I was aiming for and we discussed a few ideas. I like Keira Knightley's style in that perfume advert, but then I like a lot of things that are just not going to happen. I was kitted out with a cape, plastic shoulder mat and towel and led over to the sink where my hair was washed, conditioned, massaged and pummelled into submission. Meekly, I followed her back to the chair and read a magazine until she was finished. Couldn't look.

Finally, I had to. Hmm. Ok. It's kind of short. Oh, that's a lot of hair on the floor. But I actually like it, it swishes. I paid up and bounced out of the salon, convinced I was attracting admiring glances as I walked back to the car.

Back home, I did what every woman does after the hairdresser and raced to the biggest mirror I could find, turning this way and that, mussing it up, mentally working out if I could live with it. I think I can, although my neck's a bit cold. And I sure don't look like Keira Knightley.

8th October 2012

Doing Housework the MS Way

I used to be a real neat-freak, probably a hangover from my tiny 1-room box in London years ago, when the sofa was next to the cooker and I could switch the kettle on from my bed.

I lived there until I was 8 months pregnant and could clean the shower by simply rubbing soap on my stomach and turning round.

Up until a year ago I was still pretty much the same until jaw-dropping fatigue hit me like a demolition wrecking ball. Standards had to slide, but rather than becoming depressed, I just came up with some handy hints, which I'm now passing on to you:

- Rip up your carpets and put down wooden flooring wherever possible, adding a few non-fluffy rugs if necessary. Majorly cuts down on dirt.
- Chuck out most of your knick-knacks and ornaments – pesky dust traps.
- Use paper plates whenever you can; there's some great designs.
- Use make-up remover wipes, then when you're brushing your teeth use wipe to quickly clean sink. A bit icky, but small gestures count.

- Fit dimmers to your lights and adjust accordingly - the less dust you see, the less it matters.
- Borrow a small child. Put a feather duster in one of their hands and a lollipop in the other. Make up a fun game, but check they dust with the right one.
- Invest in light-coloured furniture (IKEA, I salute you) - shows up way less dust.
- If you *must* invite friends round, wait 'til it's dark and light candles. Lots of them. And make sure there's wine. Nothing matters after a couple of glasses.
- If questioned by worried, well-meaning friends about the shabby state of your house, simply explain you are channeling the vintage, boho-chic vibe.

William Morris once said, 'have nothing in your house that you do not know to be useful, or believe to be beautiful'. And don't forget, experts reckon a little dirt is good for your immune system, so **don't** feel guilty - you're actually looking after yourself.

12th October 2012

Oh, So I'm Ill Then?

An odd thing happened to me at my latest blood test. I have blood tests every month, so no news there. But this time, I had a new nurse.

She must have been reading my notes before she called me, as she came through to the waiting room, gently tapped me on the shoulder and gestured for me to follow. Puzzled, I put away my book and went with her. In her room, she pulled out a chair and almost helped me to sit down.

I was starting to get a bit worried. Did she know something I didn't? She sat down, clicked through her computer screen, then turned to me with big, doleful eyes and said, 'you poor, poor thing. You're what (looking back to screen), only ten years younger than me, but you're so, so brave, so strong'.

Huh? 'Oh, we don't see many people with MS here'. She asked me how I was coping with the diagnosis, what my fears for the future were and whether I had to make any...adjustments.

This got me thinking. I've been through a horrendous year and the diagnostic process isn't easy. There's no single test, there's a set of criteria you have to tick before you move from a 'single' attack to 'multiple' sclerosis.

It's incredible what you can come to think of as your new normals and you just shift your life around them. I think I'm doing pretty well and I don't live my life as an MS victim/sufferer, I just happen to have MS.

But things like this pull you up short, and the fear rises again. I really *am* ill? Finally, she took my blood pressure. 'Mm, it's awfully high. Are you anxious about anything?' Not before I came in here, I wasn't....

13th October 2012

The Kids are All Right

The Teenager is going out to a birthday party tonight. Not so very long ago, parties were held during daylight hours, the kids were exhausted from bouncing around giant soft play shapes and they had dinky party bags to take home.

Recently, parties meant a child inviting two or three close friends, taking them to a child-friendly restaurant for tea and staying with them the whole time, then embarrassing them by having the waiters bring out a birthday cake.

Now, heading for 14, the kids want to invite four or five close friends and be left, all on their own, in a restaurant for dinner. Can they even be trusted to behave? Should I follow them in disguise or wait outside in the car with binoculars? How will their waitress cope? I've seen these kids on the rugby pitch and they are LOUD. And still laugh hysterically at rude words.

The Teenager had already planned his outfit by Monday. It's been washed, ironed and hung up in his wardrobe - Fred Perry top, Next chinos. With Vans shoes. He's actually going to use deodorant and style his hair. I won't be able to get into the bathroom for at least an hour.

What should I do then? Well, I guess what any parent starved of babysitters does - head for the nearest place that sells wine. A good friend is in town, there are three pubs within walking distance of my house, I'm in remission of sorts and it's the weekend.

The kids will be fine. Luckily, I'm a cheap date now - MS has somehow made alcohol much...stronger. A couple of drinks and I'm ready to flop. And I can always blame my unbalanced walking to the loo on the MS...

16th October 2012

Pink With Envy?

I am loathe to admit it, but I used to be envious of the publicity given to breast cancer awareness - the girly sponsored walks, the dizzying range of pink goods flooding the shops every October and the endless celebrity endorsements.

By comparison, multiple sclerosis seems a very poor cousin indeed. Would it be easier for me, and society as a whole, to accept my multiple sclerosis if it was dressed up in loving, pink fluffiness? Or if I knew that thousands and thousands of strangers were doing their bit for a charity that would benefit *me*?

Yet, people are now starting to question the dubious ways in which very tenuously-linked items are being marketed to raise money for breast cancer. Recent examples include a Pink Ribbon Barbie, pink hair straighteners and a pink Makita drill, and this is only the tip of the iceberg. Are we now reaching pink overkill?

It's a contentious subject. If vast sums of money are generated and donated to search for a cure and fund services, who can grumble that it's all a bit too much and even a little tasteless. Perhaps though, by thrusting such private, personal 'battles' with breast cancer into the glare of publicity, this somehow demeans and cheapens individual experiences of the illness. Would I want to be implored to stand up, fight back, remain positive and all the other mantras by people who have no idea what it's really like? Probably not.

17th October 2012

Stockholm Syndrome

The end could be in sight - I had a second, very successful job interview yesterday and I can almost taste freedom. For my sanity, I *need* to get out of my current job.

Until recently, I had never experienced workplace bullying. When I informed my colleagues about my MS, I certainly didn't expect kid glove treatment or special measures, just a little understanding. I was completely unprepared for what happened next.

Bit by bit my duties were stripped from me. I was told that I could no longer drive for work, cutting me off from a large percentage of what my job actually entails. I was studiously ignored and excluded, most of my projects were shelved and backs were literally turned. Schoolgirl sniggers might sound harmless, but when executed effectively, they can be brutal.

In the blink of a diagnosis, I have been branded worthless, a waste of company resources and deemed less intelligent than before. Yet the only tangible change is that I chose to reduce my working hours (due to extreme fatigue), so that when I *was* in work, I could be as effective, if not more, than before.

What angers me most though, is that their callous and cruel actions have robbed me of the mental clarity needed to adjust to my diagnosis. I have been fighting a war on two fronts and it is clear they are hoping to make my life so unbearable that I will have no choice but to leave.

So why, on the threshold of a brighter future, do I feel nostalgic? Have I come to love my tormentors as a way of coping with the ongoing ordeal? I think I have had to believe that deep down, they are decent people, in order to force myself out of the house each morning.

Or perhaps it is just sadness, for never being allowed to reach my full potential.

In the meantime, as I wait for good news, I will cheer myself up by reading our company policy on 'Bullying and Harassment in the Workplace'. It's by far the best work of fiction I have read in a *long* time.

19th October 2012

Dodgy Hands and Wonky Feet

I've been bouncing off the walls the last couple of days. Quite literally.

It started in work, where I walked into the kitchen door three times. Just for good measure, my hands have decided to suddenly let go of things at random or not grasp them at all and my feet aren't working properly. I had a day off work yesterday, but rather than hiding away with Jeremy Kyle and the Loose Women, I pushed myself out the house and went off for some retail therapy and a determination not to let the symptoms get the better of me.

Bad idea? It started so well. I navigated the supermarket, dodging the Jenga towers of Christmas chocolate tins and super-value loo roll packs. Went to pick up my newspaper and failed four times. Looking around me, I pretended I *meant* to do it, undecided as I surely was about which paper to choose. Think it worked.

Got to the checkout where the bored girl sighed loudly as I fumbled with my purse. And fumbled. Couldn't open the darn zip or find my loyalty card.

Leaving with a heavy bag of shopping, I stumbled, knocked into the automatic doors and dropped my keys. Undefeated, and after being helped by the Big Issue seller standing outside, I made my way to the coffee shop. Deep breath.

Order a coffee and a poppy seed cake for being so brave. Turn round with my tray, shopping bag heaved onto my shoulder. I can definitely do this.

But somehow, within five minutes, a three-prams-and-a-double-buggy assault course had formed behind me. And the table I wanted was past them.

Ok. Co-ordinate feet, hold on to the tray very, very tightly and do not bounce off the cake cabinet.

I must have looked distinctly menacing and the mothers gripped their pram handles a little tighter. But I made it. I ate my cake, drank my coffee and watched the world go by. And when I got up to leave, I didn't knock anything off the table or drop my bags. But someone had definitely moved the door.

21st October 2012

How to Drink with MS

One of the more socially annoying aspects of having multiple sclerosis is that I am suddenly a *very* cheap date.

A couple of glasses of my favourite tipple, dry white wine, and I'm zooming away into oblivion. Or more often than not, maudlin and tearful. 'Why meeeeee', I'll wail, filling up my glass to the brim and wiping my smeared mascara all over my face. 'Don't wanna have MS, s'not fair'.

So, as with many other things in my life now, I have to be creative and think of new ways of doing things. I have now solved the alcohol conundrum. And I no longer argue with lamp posts.

I have cunningly switched from white wine to red. I can't drink red wine quickly, so I drink far less than I would if it were white. Clever, eh? Plus, it gives me a much more mellow feeling than white, so rather than wailing, I simply reflect upon how my life has changed. Like a proper grown up.

On Friday night, with The Teenager at a sleepover, I put this new-found knowledge to the test. My friend took me out to a lovely old gastro-pub in the countryside. We shared a bottle of red. Lovely. And we had a very grown-up sophisticated conversation, catching up on our week.

Sipping my wine thoughtfully, I made interesting and insightful comments.

At the next place, a café-slash-wine bar (car now safely deposited at home), we shared another bottle and had yet more intelligent conversation. And I even managed to go to the loo without stumbling.

Finally, we had a night-cap at a pub, sitting outside. I felt smugly superior to the clearly-drunk women staggering around, clutching glasses of white wine, yelling at passing cars.

I was feeling very proud now, and congratulated myself on being such a responsible adult. So maybe we shouldn't have popped into the late-night supermarket on the way home.

Waking up the next morning with a dry throat and slightly trembling hands, I went downstairs and found the previous night's spoils. A packet of Hallowe'en cakes, two supersize bags of crisps, an unopened bottle of red wine and an exercise magazine. Muppet.

22nd October 2012

The Joy of Meds

I've been taking Pregabalin (Lyrica) for over a year now
to help with the neuropathic pain I get from MS - the
burning/buzzing/stabbing pains in my legs, feet and just
about everywhere else.

Just for good measure, I also take Omega 3 fish oil,
Evening Primrose oil, multivitamins, vitamin B complex
and vitamin C with zinc, so I rattle around a fair bit every
morning.

A friend asked me recently what the pains felt like.
Tricky to explain. Some days it's as if I have mobile phones
strapped to my feet, set to vibrate constantly. Other days
it's just endless tingling and waves of pulsing, throbbing
pain.

Then there's the stabbing pains in my shoulders, the
twitching, the muscle ache. It can feel like my body is one
big marionette, pulled this way and that, controlled by
something much bigger than me.

At my last MS clinic appointment, the nurse
recommended the Lyrica should be increased and two days
ago I started the higher dose. There's no discernible
change as yet but I'm hopeful. Mostly the pain is a dull,
ever-present lurking shadow, following me everywhere and
I'm learning to live with it. But sometimes, I just want it to
stop, just for a little while. Even just for an hour, so I can

remember what it was like before all this started. A whole hour with no jerking, twitching, burning, stabbing, buzzing.

The biggest side effect of Lyrica for me is an increased appetite. I know, I know, I should eat more fruit, stock up on boiled eggs and always have a handful of nuts in my pocket. I really try.

According to the leaflet that comes with Lyrica, this can affect more than one person in 100. The leaflet makes for fascinating and thought-provoking reading. Lyrica's other side effects include tiredness, tingling feeling, clumsiness, tremor, lethargy, problems with balance, feeling drunk, abnormal style of walking, jerky movements, difficulty finding words, muscle twitching, muscle stiffness and slow or reduced movement of the body. Are you thinking what I'm thinking? Sounds *very* familiar...

22nd October 2012

Get Lost

And so it has come to pass. I went to work this morning and was called in to the boardroom (after I had made everyone cups of coffee, natch). Both bosses and little old me. I was told my job was no longer tenable and it was for my own good that I should leave.

Bear with me on this one. I was sacked for two reasons: First, my job is not viable any more. Thanks largely to being stealthily stripped of my duties over the last year, I agree with them on that point. Second, my 'health problems' mean I can no longer work at the office. What if I were to trip? What if I'm too tired one day?

I know this is highly illegal. I know I should fight. And I did, kind of. I asked to be allowed to stay for two months, until I found another job and to see me over Christmas. They will let me know their decision in a day or so.

One boss seemed stunned that I couldn't just go 'straight onto benefits' and even suggested the time I would now have on my hands would be a positive thing for me. A bit of space. He obviously lives in Daily Mail world where all disabled people on benefits sit back and coin it in.

I pointed out several times that I should have been offered the chance to bring a representative with me, especially as they are sacking me primarily on grounds of health and they had obviously had the whole weekend to construct a dismissal plan.

Gratifyingly, this seemed to alarm them, but it's cold comfort. I'm still waiting to hear back from my last job interview - hoping to get lucky. But for now, I'm going to take my big box of tissues, a family-sized bar of chocolate and a bottle of red wine, sit on the sofa and cry my eyes out.

24th October 2012

Confused But Elated

Boardroom, 9am, yesterday morning. The Showdown. Five minutes later, I'm in the car on the way home, blasting out music, giggling away to myself like a maniac. I am free.

I asked for two months and they said they would get back to me in the morning. They agree to my 'demands' on the understanding that I will work from home.

I am to go back in on Thursday morning to collect my belongings, pick up a memory stick full of the documents I need, give them a chance to gawp at the 'sacked' girl then leave behind that sad, sorry part of my life forever.

How do I feel? Shocked, confused, delirious with freedom from bullying. It's a truly disgusting scenario and I still find it hard to digest.

My world has opened up in a delicious way. I will no longer have to face day after day of endless criticism and exclusion. I no longer have to creep around, 'apologising' for my very existence and a diagnosis of multiple sclerosis.

Will I take it further? I'm speaking to an MS lawyer on Monday. I'm going to keep all possible avenues open. But for now, I have nine weeks of guaranteed income. I will be my own boss.

26th October 2012

So Long, Farewell....

The saga continues. Yesterday, I was to go to The Office Of Doom at 9am for one last time (hopefully) to pick up my belongings and the memory stick and finalise details of my employment and dismissal.

I'm all psyched up but I have no idea what I am going to face. I arrive early and call on the off-chance I can get this over with. No reply. Ten minutes later, one of the bosses hurtles out the door, so I go over to see what's happening.

Barely casting a glance in my direction, he shouts over his shoulder that he will call me later, he has to leave. Nice. I go home. Do I still have my job for two months? What's going on? My mum comes over for coffee. We go over every possible scenario. At half ten, I call the office. I need to get this over and done with.

The office junior picks up. I ask if I can come in. Of course I can. She sounds bemused. Everyone loves a drama. Coward that I am, I take my mum. We go armed with two bags and an attitude. The office junior is alone in the office. Apparently the boss has gone out to buy a memory stick.

I pack all my things, and while my mum makes the junior a cup of tea (!), I divert my emails, scribble a quick letter explaining I have left my ID card and could the memory stick be dropped off later. Collecting my mum from the kitchen where she is washing up and bleaching the sink, we leave, balancing a plant and two bulging bags between us. I look back, remembering the awful times.

It's history. But will the memory stick be dropped off? Am I still employed for two months as agreed? There's been no 'phone call, no recognition of my letter, or that I have been to collect my things. I feel humiliated and worthless. Am I really meant to be treated like this? But no matter what happens, I have my freedom. And dignity. Which is a lot more than can be said for them.

27th October 2012

Phew...

After waiting a whole morning, the memory stick is shoved through my letter box in a plain envelope. The boss knew I was in but couldn't be bothered/wasn't polite enough to knock the door and have a civil conversation.

No acknowledgement of my letter, of dropping my ID card off, clearing my stuff from the office. No 'hey, thanks for working for us for two years'. I can quite honestly say that I have never, ever been treated so shabbily in my whole life.

Being sacked for having MS is bad enough without all this game-playing on top of it. At least I have been polite, left without a squeak, but in my own way I have kicked ass. I defended myself in the boardroom when I was unexpectedly sacked on Monday, when the two bosses had so obviously been planning it for weeks.

I specifically told them I should have representation but was turned down. I negotiated two month's grace. I calmly collected my belongings. I kept in touch and was blanked. This has been a humdinger of a week.

I am an emotional wreck, high on coffee and stress. After a year of bullying, they got me out. I am angry, sad, grieving, furious, melancholic, all in equal measure. I need to calm down, think rationally and create a new plan. I'm struggling not to take it personally. How can I not?

Maybe the writing was on the wall when I spent a week in hospital for MS treatment over the summer, and was on sick leave for three weeks (statutory sick pay, the bare minimum). Not a Get Well Card, not a phone call or visit. No communication whatsoever.

It's the small things that hurt the most. In our little office, we buy chocolate eclairs when there is a celebration. Guess what I found in the fridge on Thursday when I was clearing out my stuff? A big box of them. Wonder what they were celebrating?

28th October 2012

A Recipe for Changing Your Life

This is best for the novice cook - the less experience you have, the better.

Ingredients

- A good few relapses - drop into mixing bowl, one after the other in rapid succession.
- One firm diagnosis of multiple sclerosis - this could take you a while to obtain, so be patient.
- Two evil bosses. If these are difficult to find, check under stones, where they're fond of crawling out from.
- A liberal sprinkling of heavy-grade bullying at work, of the nastier and more vicious variety.
- For added panache, throw in an unfair dismissal along with a copy of the Disability Discrimination Act.
- Finally, a generous dash of steroids, MRIs and a lumbar puncture.

Method

- Mix all the ingredients together well. You are aiming for a gloopy, gungy consistency
- Simmer at the highest temperature for just over a year.

Best served with

- The best friends you can find (you know who you are)
- A darn good support network - www.shift.ms and www.mssociety.org.uk are amongst the finest
- Copious amounts of chocolate and laughter

After digesting, pick yourself up, dust yourself down and get out of the kitchen. There's a bright, shiny new world waiting for you...

31st October 2012

Just Hook Me Up

I'm living on coffee and stress so why am I putting on weight?

I want to be one of these people who sheds pounds when they're dashing around like a headless chicken, pumped up with stress and an unfair dismissal.

My mind is racing, but it seems my body isn't. It's just over a week since I was sacked for having MS. There is too much to do, apart from the everyday routine, the Christmas planning, the taxi service for The Teenager. Throw in all the ubiquitous health appointments, blood tests, a newly-diagnosed day and a fatigue management course and I'm up against it.

So the thought of launching a legal case is filling me with fear, and coffee. I (think) I am a nice person. I don't like fighting. At school, I gave my lunch money to the bullies without a word. But this scenario, the one I am facing right now, is out of my league.

The bullying at work was horrendous enough. A year of loathing myself for not standing up to them, whilst battling to come to terms with my diagnosis and what it means for my future.

Perhaps there is a tipping point. By dismissing me on the spot, expecting me to clear my desk and leave straight away has made me angry. I would hate myself more for walking away. What have I got to lose? I have had incredible support. My healthcare professionals have risen up in outrage and anger, my friends have rallied round and my forum buddies have carried me along on a wave of advice and calming words.

One of them pointed out that I would only ever have to do this once. Excellent point. I *have* to do this.

3rd November 2012

Doing The Big Shop

In a bid to get my routine back on track, I got up early yesterday to go for the Big Shop. I can't seem to plan a week ahead though, so I normally just buy some meat, vegetables, pasta and rice and cobble meals together on a day-to-day basis, always having to buy extra ingredients each day.

One of my first symptoms of MS was being unable to plan *anything* at all. My brain just would not compute basic things and I got confused easily. Food shopping was a nightmare. I would stand and stare at the rows of food, unable to decide what I needed and end up grabbing random things and chucking them in my trolley.

I couldn't even follow simple recipes so we lived off baked potatoes and microwave meals for a long while. But, I was upbeat and optimistic. If I stuck to the basics, I couldn't go wrong.

I parked up, glared at the builder's van taking up two disabled spaces and marched into the store. I wandered up and down the aisles, panic rising. So many special offers, so many meal deals. Three things for a tenner, five things for a tenner, buy one, get one half price. Plus Christmas carols playing in the background.

I could feel my brain melting. As I circled the aisles again and again, I couldn't choose anything. Deep breath.

Got some salmon. Got a big bag of potatoes, some carrots, few tins of tuna. Stand for ages in front of the ten pound meal deal. Two starters, two mains, one dessert. Mathematical equation. Is it me or is it hot in here?

Finally, I make it to the till where the checkout woman chucks my food through so fast, I get nervous, drop things, can't pack the bags. Hands don't want to hold anything today, but mission is finally accomplished.

When I get home, I stagger into the house, laden with bags, rain pouring down and trip over the cat. It's bizarre how the most simple, taken-for-granted tasks can become an assault course when you have MS. I was planning to make cottage pie for dinner, but the recipe is confusing the hell out of me and I forgot the Worcestershire sauce...

5th November 2012

Rugby Mum.....And MS

I like The Teenager playing rugby. He won't mind me saying he was pretty dire to start with a couple of years ago, but he's nothing if not determined. Now, he's got real promise and has offered to buy me a luxury penthouse granny flat if he becomes famous.

Only problem is, I don't understand the game at all. Before MS, I would duly stand on the side lines, muffled in a couple of layers of jumpers, wellie boots on and teeth chattering. I took my cue from the screaming crowd, and cheered along when something happened. Sometimes for the wrong team, but never mind.

I schlepped to every game, took him to every training session and washed a pile of muddy clothes twice a week. We even went 'on tour' last year, aka an excuse for the parents to let the kids run wild while we got blind, steaming drunk. So drunk, I was nominated to go first on the karaoke, where I sang 'Gold' atrociously and still got applauded.

This was right before my first major relapse and there was an inkling there was something wrong when I went bright red in the face after a leisurely stroll and my legs turned to jelly.

So now, post-MS, the rugby routine is a little different. I still take him training and I still wash his kit but there's no way I can go to every game. I can't stand up for long, I'm normally tired beyond belief and my legs get too weak.

If there's an away game, I have to ask for The Teenager to have a lift as I don't drive too far - my foot cramps up. Which is awkward, as every time I see one of the rugby parents, they scrutinise me closely, look me up and down and say, 'But you look so...well?' A code phrase for, 'lazy cow, any excuse, eh?'

Yesterday, the game was cancelled as the pitch is saturated with rain. Am I unhappy? What do you think?

9th November 2012

Magical Alemtuzumab

The day I was diagnosed with MS, my neurologist told me that mine was the highly-active or rapidly-evolving sort. I had two choices. The usual disease-modifying drugs such as Copaxone or Rebif or I could choose Alemtuzumab (Campath).

It's a drug used to treat leukaemia, and in laywoman's terms, it strips out your immune system, killing the T-cells involved in the MS immune response. There's some pretty serious side-effects including a 1 in 3 chance of developing a thyroid problem, but it can halt the progression of MS for at least 10 years by reducing the number of relapses. A no-brainer for me - I was having relapse after relapse with barely time to catch my breath in between.

It was like being thrown against a wall repeatedly. My body was battered and bruised, I couldn't walk properly, I slept all the time and fell over a lot. So, it was an easy choice and I know just how fortunate I was.

Alemtuzumab is still unlicensed for use with MS, but was given to me off licence. All I wanted was to be able to see The Teenager off to university in a couple of years. I didn't want him to be my carer, or always to be too tired to take him anywhere.

After five days in hospital, hooked up to an IV, pumped full of chemicals and steroids, I was back home without an immune system for the next few weeks. Now, four months on, a miracle has taken place. I still get tired but I don't need to sleep the afternoon away, I haven't fallen over, I can walk (stumble) far better than before and I just generally feel, well, normal(ish) again.

I haven't had a relapse...yet. Touch wood. Don't walk on cracks on the pavement. I still have a whole bag of symptoms, just not all at once. A novel experience.

12th November 2012

Relapse Hide and Seek

Most of us with relapsing-remitting MS will be familiar with examining every tiny little symptom and asking, 'is *this* a relapse or am I just being over-sensitive/paranoid?'. We live in constant fear and easily forget how, pre-MS, we got sick anyway and sometimes we felt under par or just generally a bit rubbish.

Post-MS, the situation shifts. A relapse is Bad News. They can last for as little as a few days or for as long as several months and initially the symptoms can be confusing. I can quite honestly say, I have never analysed my health in so much ridiculously fine detail.

I wake up every morning and lie there for a little while mentally scanning through my body. How do I feel? Anything odd? Ok, get out of bed. How's my balance? Am I a bit more wibbly on my feet than usual? Standing in the shower, can I raise my hands ok? It is *constant*.

One day, I woke up from an afternoon nap in blind terror. My left hand was numb. I couldn't move it at all and I began to panic - how would I change gears in the car, how could I go shopping with a dud hand? You can imagine how stupid I felt when I realised I had slept on it.

So I play a constant game of relapse hide and seek. If I pretend there's nothing really wrong, well, there's nothing really wrong, is there? I'll just stay one step ahead of the game. MS is like a constant heat-seeking missile, on the prowl, stalking you all the time.

Just for fun, you can also have a pseudo-relapse, a temporary flare up, commonly triggered by stress, heat or exertion. I think this is what happened to me last week. I had a friend over for wine and a gossip, but I felt odd (*before* the bottle was opened....) - a spaced-out feeling I normally get at the start of a relapse.

I tried to shrug it off and laugh about it, but in the back of my mind, I was running away and hiding. Fast. Luckily, it came to nothing and I woke up fine the next day. For now then, I am relapse-free and I hope to remain so for a good time yet. Until we meet again, Mr Relapse, go away and leave me in peace....

13th November 2012

Fatigue Management for the Weary

I was invited to join an MS Fatigue Management course, which started yesterday. The aim is to discuss strategies for coping with fatigue, the impact it can have and to meet people in a similar situation.

Our little gang is now proud to be launching a new campaign - to redefine MS fatigue/tiredness/exhaustion as 'Clinical Fatigue', in the hope that we will be taken more seriously.

Fatigue is one of the most common symptoms in MS and around 80% of us have it. There is a medical reason for it, called demyelination. Nerves are covered in a coating or sheath called myelin. If that gets damaged the nerves are exposed. Literally, bad nerves. Result, progressive MS. Ok, technical bit over, now the day-to-day reality.

MS fatigue is like being run over by a big lorry of tiredness and squashed flat. It can strike out of nowhere. It can seriously get in the way of life and is similar to how you would feel if you were awake for 48 hours non-stop. So why the song and dance?

Well, it's just so *darned* difficult to convey to friends, family, work, random strangers that this is *extreme* tiredness. Off the scale in intensity. Typical conversation:

Them: *How are you today (looking me up and down). You look good?*

Me: *Oh, I'm cream-crackered. Exhausted.*

Them: *Yeah, know just how you feel. I was pooped last night.*

Me: *No, I mean really, really tired.*

Them: *God, yeah. That's like me every day. But you look so well!*

Me: *I'm off to bed...ta ra.*

It's frustrating. I would bang my head against the wall in frustration if it didn't make me so tired, and anyhow, there's enough damage in my brain already.

The course was excellent and I met some brilliant people. It's refreshing to hear that I'm not making it up, the tiredness is not me being lazy. This is why we want to campaign to redefine MS fatigue, give it a proper, medical name. So from now on, we will be referring to it as 'Clinical Fatigue', to give it the gravitas it deserves. I would go out with a placard and march up and down the street, but I am exhausted and I'm going to squeeze in a quick nap before The Teenager gets back from school.

14th November 2012

Working from Home (Alone)

So, I get sacked from work for having MS and negotiate a two-month notice period working from home to get my finances in order and find a new job. In theory (forget the unfair dismissal and discrimination), it's great. A bit of breathing space, a chance to get my head together and move on.

In reality, it's hard. I miss the buzz of getting up and out the house, feeling like a valuable member of society. I miss my work wardrobe, even though it had shrunk to only black clothes in the last few months, reflecting the depression I was sinking into at work. And I miss packing a little lunch into my work bag. Hell, I even miss making coffee for the others in the office.

To shake things up a little, I decided to go to the local mega-supermarket to check out the end-of-aisle bargains. I left the house early, pretending to be a commuter. Parked up, picked up a basket and started having a nosy around, ending up in the towel and shower curtain aisle by mistake. Seems the mega-superstore had been given a major refurb without consulting me and half the aisles were now diagonal, not straight. How to confuse an idiot, eh?

So I pick up some mushrooms, 2-for-1 pasta, a pack of reduced turkey mince and a value pack of toothbrushes - well worth leaving the house for. I get home, have a cup of coffee with the cat and sit down at my desk again. Right.

Work like a demon for a couple of hours, check on Twitter, then it's lunch. Sit down with the Loose Women. Then back to work. It's a pretty lonely day. All my friends are in their proper jobs, the mummies in the cafés won't talk to me (where can I borrow a baby from?) and the postman hasn't time to stop for a chat.

I can't wait to work with other people again. I will fling myself gratefully upon them, greeting them like long-lost friends. I will bring a box of doughnuts in every Friday. In the meantime though, it's amazing what you can make from office supplies, isn't it? To cheer myself up, I string paperclips together (festive), cut sticky smiley faces from post-it notes (funny) and make little monsters from mini-clips (strangely sad). I think it's time I found myself a proper job.

18th November 2012

In A&E - But Not For Me

Strange to be on the other side of the sick bed. My friend was visiting when he started having terrible stabbing and tingling pains over half his face, along with a pressure headache and a painful eye. Hmm, sounding slightly neurological, no?

After a bit of kerfuffle ('I'm not sick, me man, we are strong'), I managed to drag/push him through the doors of our local A&E, marched him up to the desk and got him booked in. We got seen pretty quickly, a huge range of tests were carried out, he was prodded and poked and we speedily googled everything they told us.

I had great fun pulling the ECG tabs from his chest and when the lunch trolley came round, we shared some corned beef and pickle sandwiches, chatted away and tried to stay calm. Hospitals are funny places. All human life is here.

In the opposite cubicles, a man was lying all on his own, the man next to him was having his arm put back into its socket and there was a tiny lady with wispy hair wandering around talking to everyone about her walking stick and a suit she should have been wearing (no, me neither).

I clearly remember being in the same assessment unit, just over a year ago. I was frightened and in a state of shock. I had booked myself in because I woke up and couldn't speak properly - mixing up words, unable to find the right word, generally talking more rubbish than usual. All this made me feel kind of thankful that the whole diagnostic process was now behind me. After a year of tests, knock-backs, uncertainty and fear, yes, I have MS. But at least I know what I am dealing with.

Within a couple of hours, the doctor decided my friend wasn't having a stroke or suffering from anything seriously neurological, it was an episode of trigeminal neuralgia. Painful but treatable. We collected his prescription and left. It was good to feel useful in an emergency and for it not always to be about me. He is now resting at home. I hope. Knowing him, he'll be back at work. Oi, if you're reading this, get back on that sofa and look after yourself - you never know when I might need your help again....

19th November 2012

Walking Stick Chic

Gandalf has one, Charlie Chaplin was famous for his and Brad Pitt was recently spotted with one. So why am I so reluctant to use a walking stick when I need to?

This came up for discussion last week in the Fatigue Management course, when I wailed about how scary it was to walk to the loo in a busy pub or restaurant (I have been known to trip and fall spectacularly, in full cartoon-mode). I can sit there for hours, carefully plotting the best route, working out how slippery the floor is and counting how many people I could quite possibly fall over in front of.

If I don't know where the loos are, I will send a friend first and extract every last bit of information from them. 'How far did you say? Big plant to watch out for? Carpet or wooden flooring?'. And so on.

The suggestion from the group was that I should carry one of those folding ones in my bag and just use it for extra balance when I need to. It's a huge psychological step though, isn't it?

It's almost the same as the first time you go outside with a pram - you think everyone is looking at you and it takes a while to get used to it. And how on earth do you actually walk with it? I think I may need a few trial runs. I will go out when it is dark, in dark clothing to a very dark place and give it a go. Do you put the stick down first, then walk or walk then put the stick down? What's the rhythm? What if I trip over the stick?

I had a chat with a friend a while back about this conundrum. She put her hand on my arm and said, 'Daaaarling (she's a bit posh), never fear! Why do you think all the best ballet teachers have one? It gives them authority, it is chic and makes a statement'. Fair point.

So the last time I was in town, I scanned the crowds, picking out every single person with a stick. I failed to find a single chic person. The majority were eligible for free bus passes. Where are all the young people with sticks? Where do they hide?

21st November 2012

The Christmas Work Party...For One

A delicious thought struck me the other day. This year, for the first time in well over a decade, I will not be going to a Christmas work party.

Technically I am still employed until the end of December, but I'm guessing I'd be as welcome as a new lesion on an MRI scan.

This means I won't spend days (weeks) agonizing over my party outfit, striking the right balance between chic and trashy. I won't need to find a 'jolly' pair of flashing Christmas tree earrings, or drape tinsel round my neck and I won't need to get involved in a Secret Santa present-swap, so no sneaky trip to Poundland then (I highly recommend the candles and picture frames - wrapped in expensive paper, who'd know?).

Most of the work parties in recent years have been excruciating exercises in 'office bonhomie'. The boss is generally dressed down in dodgy 'cool' clothes, they've put twenty quid behind the bar and we all sit there with a limp cracker and a single party popper.

Conversation stumbles along until enough cheap alcohol is consumed and it's at this point that all hell usually lets loose. Old resentments spring up, snarky comments are traded and the boss just sits there, eyes glazed, trying to get us all to tell rude jokes.

Inevitably, one or more of the women will rush to the loo, crying, followed by a gaggle of other women, eager to be the first with the gossip. With Christmas carols playing on a loop in the background, one or two will attempt to grab random drunken men for a dance and the smokers will decamp with their drinks to the back terrace and remain there the rest of the evening.

Am I sad then, to be missing out on all this fun? Er, no. It's a relief. So I have decided to throw my own party for one. I'll go to Waitrose for a nice selection of party nibbles, pour some Cava, put Cliff Richard's Christmas CD on and have a fabulous time.

There'll be no need to dress up, so I'll have a 'pyjama party' dress code. There'll be no embarrassing photographs being emailed round the following morning unless the cat has developed opposable thumbs and there will be a sense of relief not to go to the office the next day only to be met with raised eyebrows. So, to all of you who have an office party to go to, good luck and raise a glass to me...I'll be thinking of you.

25th November 2012

Happy Anniversary, MS (you suck)

Hey, MS, Happy 6 Month Anniversary! After a year of hell, I was officially diagnosed on 25th May.

I don't need to tell most of you how horrendous the diagnostic process can be, suffice to say I am overjoyed never, ever to have to go through a lumbar puncture again. Have you *seen* those needles?

Having MS sweep into your life is like having an ugly, unwanted house-guest move in with two huge suitcases and the kitchen sink. For ever. No matter how much you try to get on with life, work around them and keep ignoring them in the hope they will go away, they stick around.

Not content with that, they inflict pain on you mercilessly in unexpected ways, physically, mentally and emotionally. They rack up extra costs, they stop you going out as much as before and they chuck out your heels (that was a cheap, low shot, MS). They rob you of your health, your confidence and your zest. They frighten your family and taunt you about your diminishing prospects.

If MS were a person, they'd be arrested and banged up for life. So how do I feel, six months on? The absolute permanence of MS horrifies me. It will never go away. The progression of it, too, is something I tuck away in the furthest reaches of my mind, only to be thought about in very dark moments. I hate the constant fear, the gnawing anxiety of a relapse just around the corner.

I hate the way MS has shaken my life so completely to its foundations that nothing is the same as before. I know, I need to *embrace* this illness. I should accept that MS is now indelibly imprinted on my life. I need to Think Positive! Meditate, do yoga, give up the sweets, the alcohol, the stress. Don't we all?

If pushed, I would say that the one thing MS has given me is the ability to appreciate things more. Not in a hippy-dippy, mung-bean eating way - just enjoying small pockets of time when everything is ok. I don't take so much for granted now.

I'm still debating whether to get a tattoo to mark this little anniversary. Something small, just between me and MS. I want a barcode, with the words, Best Before 25/05/12. Or should that be Best After...?

26ᵗʰ November 2012

Christmas All Wrapped Up

Well, possible relapse to one side, I am sadly excited to report I have Christmas all wrapped up. This time last year, I was 'lucky'. I was on my second course of steroids for yet another relapse and I was flying.

I couldn't sleep, I had extreme amounts of energy and I was absolutely buzzing. I would wake at 4am every morning and, possessed with a demon drive, I wouldn't get to sleep 'til gone midnight. My house has never been so clean - all that energy had to go somewhere. The lightbulbs were dusted, the skirting boards scrubbed and every single bit of cutlery cleaned to within an inch of its life.

I put the tree up one morning at 5am. It was fully decorated and lit by 6am. I whizzed around supermarkets, wrote endless lists and had everything planned with military precision.

Only problem was, once the steroids had left my system, I was a rag doll, limp and lifeless, with a fixed grin on my face. This year, I have fulfilled my steroid quota, so no bonus energy for me. With that in mind, I *need* to get Christmas sorted, just in case.

So yesterday, I finished my present shopping, chose wrapping paper and tasteful ribbon and even rounded the trip off with a quick visit to Starbucks, The Teenager in tow. I had bribed him with a chocolate shortbread and one of those strawberry drinks with squirty cream on top.

This Christmas, the theme in my house is 'Scandinavian Minimalism', cleverly hiding the fact I have no energy to loop endless decorations onto a huge tree. I bought two small trees and decorated them simply, with lots of white lights and nothing else.

I found a sculpture of a reindeer made from driftwood and will be wearing a Sarah Lund jumper for most of December. I will disguise my tiredness with Nordic gloominess and a contemplative demeanour. Meatballs and cloudberry juice will be served, along with almond biscuits and salted liquorice.

One thought keeps recurring though. Can I save up my steroid quota next year and use them at Christmas? Mandatory steroids for all those with MS! A new campaign? Right, where's the Akavit? God Jul!

29th November 2012

Needle Fiddle Faddle

Until my epidural, needles held no fear for me, but trying to stay completely still whilst being racked by labour pains is no laughing matter.

I swore off needles for life, there and then. Ha! Now it seems needles feature quite a lot in my life, another side-effect, brought to me courtesy of MS and yesterday I was off to the surgery for another blood test.

Last year, on the basis of a suspect MRI, I was whisked off for a lumbar puncture. People are divided about these. Some have great experiences and sail through them, tutting loudly and wondering what all the fuss is about at us lot who scream their way through them.

It wasn't the doctor's fault that he'd never done one before. The needle (huge, vile thing) kept hitting bone. No words could possibly begin to describe the pain.

Over an hour later, I loosened the grip on my mum's hand, tears pouring down my face, in absolute agony. And if I thought that was horrific enough, worse was to come. The skull-crushing lumbar puncture headache. It lasted a week. It literally (and I don't use that word lightly), felt like my brain was being squeezed. Probably the most painful experience of my life *ever*.

This summer, whilst in hospital having Alemtuzumab treatment for MS, I had a cannula inserted and it was to stay in my hand for a week. A week! I managed four days until it fell off in the shower, recreating a massacre scene, blood spurting everywhere.

As part of the monitoring process, I have to have a full blood count taken every month for five years, plus I'm due my second and hopefully last course of Alemtuzumab next year. I'm an old hand at this now - every time I see a doctor or nurse, I automatically roll up my sleeve. Is it slightly sad though, to be disappointed not to get a sticker for being so brave?

3rd December 2012

Woo Hoo! (Possibly, Maybe)

I woke up yesterday morning and felt strange.

I had a shower, made coffee, put the cat out and still felt strange. I had....energy. How bizarre. Where did that come from?

After a couple of weeks of feeling punch-drunk with tiredness, this was altogether frightening as well as exhilarating. How long will it last? How many things can I cram into this window of opportunity?

I have to calm down and think straight. I rummaged round in the kitchen drawer and pulled out my list of 'Things To Do When I'm Not Tired'. I scanned through it. None of them will happen.

I'm definitely not climbing a ladder to get the leaves out of the guttering. With my balance? And I won't be painting the bedroom doors - what if I get hit with fatigue half-way through? The doors could remain semi-painted for weeks, months.

So my revised tick-list is a little less ambitious. Cook dinners from scratch, vacuum through whole house (not just the bits I can see), sort out accounts, shred that pile of old paperwork and get rid of the cobwebs that have been tormenting me from the sofa.

The thing with MS fatigue is, when the door of energy opens, you have no idea whatsoever how long it will be before it slams shut again. A day? A week? My mind was buzzing. So many things to choose from. I could watch a complicated, subtitled film and actually follow it, I could attempt to cook a mushroom Wellington, I could dust off my Nordic ski poles and go walking.

I spent most of the day doing almost nothing, paralysed with indecision yet marvelling at actually having energy and a clear head. I read half a book, as I had the energy to concentrate and not drift off. I wrote more lists of things I have to do. I caught up with my emails.

I know I should have done a whole lot more, but I was just enjoying the sensation of being fully awake. The fact that I *could* do things if I chose to was enough for me. Being able to think straight without my head being full of cotton wool gave me a chance to get my head in order. I have a busy week ahead. I'm hoping to keep the energy going and tick some more things off my list. Give me a break, eh, MS?

4th December 2012

I'm Still Going...

Well, this is fabulous. The energy levels are holding up and I feel on top of the world.

A lot of my ongoing symptoms seem to be disappearing too, except for the numb left arm. But hey, I still have the other one. The only drawback is that I woke up ultra early. So early, even the cat didn't come downstairs for another hour.

After getting nothing done the day before, I whizzed through a couple of hours of work, put a load of laundry on, plumped up the sofa cushions, rearranged the food cupboards and watered the plants.

At 7am I woke The Teenager with a cheery yell but judging by the grunts coming from under the duvet, he wasn't feeling quite as awake as I was. But the sun was shining and I looked back on my recent fatigue with a shudder.

You don't realise just how awful it is until it's over. So tedious, so mind-numbingly boring and depressing. I know this might not last though, so I am laying down plans for how to cope the next time the fatigue juggernaut rolls around: The sofa becomes the centre of operation. Therefore it is vital to have everything within easy reach.

It's amazing just how much you can get done whilst lying down - emails, paperwork, phone calls, Twitter. Must make sure I have remote control to hand, that there's a good stack of programmes on Sky Planner (nothing too taxing - Come Dine With Me, Escape to the Country and America's Next Top Model), a couple of magazines and a generous supply of snacks.

With a bit of luck, you can also socialise from your sofa. Invite a friend over and casually suggest they swing by the takeaway. If you've got a teensy bit of energy but not enough to go out on a Friday night, have a friend over for a bottle of wine. Stay on the sofa, but prop yourself up (you don't want to seem rude). When they leave, just slide back down and resume resting position. Simples.

5th December 2012

Because I Said So

'In my day' are words I *never* thought I would say. But I do, a lot. As well as 'when I was your age' and 'because I said so'.

When did this happen? It all makes me feel rather...old. When I was pregnant, I swore that I would never turn into a boring old parent. I would be cool and trendy (these words alone are a dead giveaway of my age).

I would give my child freedom to express themselves, to follow their own dream all the while gently nudging them along the right path. Then he turned into The Teenager and I find myself trudging the same old path as my mum did.

The Teenager and I communicate in single sentences. I say, 'put your coat on, you'll get cold', 'turn that racket down', 'close the fridge, you're wasting energy' and 'I gave you coat hangers for a reason'. He normally replies, 'yeah, whatever' with exaggerated rolling of the eyeballs.

One day I asked him to turn off his computer and get on with some homework only to be met with 'like, duh, I'm just emailing it to my teacher.' Huh?' I told him 'in my day the internet didn't exist'. He looked momentarily stunned. Wide-eyed, he asked me how I survived, did we have Sky Planner, how did we meet up with friends?

Yup, I felt practically prehistoric, a dinosaur. Now we have MS in the equation, it's slightly tricky to get the balance right. I make up for the bad days with treats. The chip shop will no doubt be sending me a Christmas card this year.

I buy little cakes for after school, I let him have more sleepovers than usual and I still wash his rugby boots even though he's old enough to do it himself. I don't want him to feel his childhood is overshadowed by MS, and fortunately for me a lot of my symptoms are invisible. So for now, we are trucking along just fine. Now if you'll excuse me, I'm just off to settle down with my People's Friend and a cup of tea. Ooh, and a nice Garibaldi biscuit. Lovely.

7th December 2012

But You Look So Well

Five words guaranteed to raise the blood pressure of us 'invisible' MSers, 'but you look so well' is normally accompanied by a sharply raised eyebrow and a sceptical look.

Obviously I've been making the whole sorry saga up and have accepted help and sympathy under false pretences. The meaning behind these words is stark: you said you were ill, but you're clearly not. Go away, you attention-seeking drama queen.

I get asked to explain my symptoms. Dodgy balance, extreme fatigue, wonky hands, difficulty walking in a straight line, falling over. They nod then say, 'well, at least it's not cancer, eh, bet you're glad it's nothing more serious?'

There is an illness hierarchy and MS languishes somewhere near the bottom. Sure, on the surface I do look fine, and since being diagnosed with MS, it's important to me to still look my best. Adapting to the role of a 'sick person' has been a difficult transition and one I am still going through. Yet, for society to regard you as an ill person or a person with a disability, you need to conform to their expectations, otherwise you may as well whistle for support.

I should stop washing, start wearing baggy-kneed leggings bought in bulk from Primark, rub chip-fat into my hair and under no circumstances dare to put even the merest hint of make-up on.

I must give up work, apply to go on the Jeremy Kyle show and start hanging out in Poundland, spending my benefits on cheap junk food. A well-meaning friend joked that MS fatigue is a pretty cushy symptom; you get to doss around on the sofa all day, doing nothing more taxing than changing the telly channel.

What they don't see is the fear, the anxiety and the utter terror of an uncertain future. MS is sneaky. Its symptoms can strike at any time and there's no set pattern. You can be chatting away in Starbucks, feeling quite normal, enjoying your latte when suddenly the cup drops from your hand. Or you can be walking along the street when your foot just gives way from under you.

Socially, MS is dire. It steals your confidence. So if you see a person with MS looking well, just think of the effort they've made despite everything. And don't mention the Poundland carrier bag full of Frey Bentos pies and Bacon Bite crisps...

8th December 2012

MRI...Meh

I had a neurology appointment yesterday, to check how I'm getting on since the Alemtuzumab treatment I had in the summer.

I always arrive early at hospital to have a wander round the shops in the main concourse and chill with a (revolting) coffee and a spot of people-watching.

I bought some bits and pieces from Boots, including an horrendously overpriced Jamie Oliver sandwich then wandered over to the gift /clothing shop. Who goes to hospital and buys cruise-wear? Or a new handbag? I decided against buying a new sparkly, spangly scarf and went to W H Smiths instead and looked at the expensive books.

Anyway, I had some coffee with my mum and watched the clock tick round before heading off to the clinic. The appointment went well, although I had to go through those neurological tests again - you know, the ones similar to the tests American cops make you do when they stop people for drink-driving; touch your nose with your finger and walk in a straight line heel-to-toe. Luckily, I am normal - and not drunk - and didn't fall over or make a fool of myself. However, the bad news is that I will need to have another MRI scan next year.

If I had to choose between an hour-long lumbar puncture and an MRI, I would choose a lumbar puncture any day. I absolutely loathe small spaces. I am claustrophobic beyond all reason.

When I was a kid, my sister locked me in a wardrobe, went for lunch and forgot all about me. Pot-holing as a hobby fills me with horror. I've had two MRIs and have no idea how I got through them. You're given earplugs, fitted with a guard to keep your head still and told you can keep your eyes open and look in the mirror set above you. Er, not a chance. My eyes were squeezed shut the entire time.

You go in head first and it is terrifying. The magnets whizz round making a racket and it's freezing cold. Each time, I could feel blind panic rising and each time I moved my mind to a happy place, anywhere rather than in that Tube of Terror.

So I have seven months to prepare. I will do my yogic breathing exercises, employ visualisation techniques and pretend I am lying on a very cold, hard beach.

14th December 2012

Retail Therapy

Another day on the MS rollercoaster. To add to the long list of weird and wonderful symptoms MS has given me, I have just experienced vertigo for the first time.

It started two days ago and I still have it, but I had to go Christmas shopping with my mum yesterday. I finally decided against wearing black to the Christmas Day lunch, so I thought a cheery, berry-red sparkly top would be perfect and we went to town to find one.

First mistake was getting a bus. When you can't move your head without it spinning, it's hard to sit still on a packed bus as it bounced over every pothole, swung sharply round corners and took a roundabout at top speed. Second mistake was assuming that as it was Christmas, the shops would be filled with cheery, berry-red sparkly tops.

There were lots and lots of black tops, black sparkly tops and black lacy tops. Lots of hideous prints. No velvet tops, which was odd. The only red tops I could find were either prim, buttoned-up cardigans or sheer, floaty ones which would reveal far too much of my muffin-top. Nothing cheery and sparkling.

We went in and out of most of the shops on the high street and eventually I found a cream sparkly top. Result! I also treated myself to a necklace with a single silver star on it. Now I'm all ready for the big day, but the jury's still out on whether I should accessorise with reindeer antlers or flashing Christmas tree earrings.

My mum bought me a Sarah Lund-ish jumper for Christmas(all the badgering paid off) and I cheered myself up with some goodies from Waitrose. Then, a stroke of luck - as we were headed back to the bus stop, laden down with bags, my builder friend was working nearby and offered us a lift home.

We must have looked a right pair, cramming my mum's shopping trolley and four large carrier bags into the back of his van but we managed it. Anyway, the vertigo is still here and it's the oddest thing.

Everything spins and I feel constantly dizzy and ill. The only way I can get any relief is to lie down. That's not really practical when I've still got work to do, so I've been bravely battling on. If I can just put in another few hours, I have a huge bag of chocolate toffees to chomp on later. And I can definitely eat them lying down, with my eyes closed.

19th December 2012

Eat, Don't Eat

Do you know what really, really annoys me about Christmas time? We're encouraged to stuff our faces, over-indulge, drink too much, inhale whole tins of Roses and slump on the sofa all day long. Which is lovely. I don't need an excuse at all.

But isn't it *so* annoying to pick up the newspapers on Boxing Day only be told off for our over-excess and shouldn't we think about dieting? Make your mind up.

I am loving this week before the Big Day. My social diary is full, I'm catching up with my long-neglected friends and the usual timetable is suspended. There's expectation in the air.

We've reached the fag-end of the year and it's time to reflect and move forward, fuelled by chocolate and mince pies. Come the weekend, it will be totally acceptable to have a glass or two of mulled wine in the afternoon, and if I feel like dropping off in front of the telly, I can. Then I'll pour myself a Bailey's - only at Christmas - and decide what else to eat.

Boxing Day will bring me back to earth with a thud. Magazines and newspapers flood into the newsagents, full of diets, rebukes and remorse. My local gym will hang up banners chiding me for my gluttony, offering me a free towel if I'm one of the first 50 to sign up for their overpriced membership. Can't we just enjoy a week or two of sheer indulgence without the shame afterwards?

It's exactly the same every year. It's the same with the sun-drenched holiday adverts that pop up on telly. We're deep in the middle of Christmas, we don't want to be thinking about booking our next holiday. We're praying for a little bit of snow. Can't you wait until mid-January? Christmas isn't over yet. I just want a chance to relax and enjoy myself.

I still haven't lost the weight I put on with the steroids I took for three different MS relapses, so give me a break. If I want to buy a Family Circle box of biscuits and eat them all by myself while watching The Sound of Music for the 27th time, I will. I can blame MS. It's a great excuse.

21st December 2012

The End of The World or a New Beginning?

This could very well be my last ever blog post if the Mayans are correct. I haven't managed to stockpile supplies for the forecast apocalypse. It's been difficult enough buying in extra food for Christmas, so if it does happen and we somehow survive, we'll be living on shortbread, Ferrero Rocher and white wine for the next week or so until the Co-op re-opens.

Assuming the apocalypse doesn't go ahead as planned, today is a significant day. It is the winter solstice. I won't be heading to Stonehenge in a flowing skirt decorated with bells and crystals, but I do think it's a pretty special time.

It's the shortest day of the year, the slide into darkness is at an end and symbolically, this means an awful lot to me. Today is my last day in my old job and the less said about that, the better. The solstice represents a rebirth, a renewal of sorts. The period of mourning for my old life, old job, old plans is now drawing to a close.

I am buzzing with ideas and my confidence has been slowly rebuilt after being eroded by others over the last year. Life is looking brighter than it has in a long time. I have been working from home for the last two months and for the last couple of weeks I have not done any housework bar the absolute minimum.

Not because I'm a lazy cow (honest), but as a symbol of new beginnings, I am going to clean my house from top to bottom today. No more working from home, the house will once again be reclaimed as a sanctuary.

I'm going to fling all the windows and doors open and let fresh air flood in. If it wasn't raining, I would hang the duvets from the windows like they do in Switzerland, but a good fluffing will have to do.

Today, then, marks the start of my new life. If I wake up on Saturday morning and the world is still here, watch out, because I've got my sassy pants on...

27TH December 2012

Excess All Areas

Well, I have had an excellent Christmas. It may be getting harder to squeeze into my jeans, but you can't go to a family get together and nibble on celery sticks, can you?

I have eaten thousands and thousands of calories over the last few days and have enjoyed every single one of them. The Teenager rolled up his sleeves and helped serve Christmas lunch to forty-odd pensioners on Christmas Day, bless him. He was a bit shy to start with, but got into his stride and was soon happily scooting round, doling out roast potatoes, slices of turkey and carrots.

Everyone agreed that he was 'a very nice young man, very nice, and ooh, so tall, what was I feeding him, Baby Bio?' There was only one awkward moment. We all had to gather in the hall and sing along to carols. A woman went round with a box full of musical instruments and feeling very Christmassy, I grabbed a couple of plastic maracas and enthusiastically shook them along to 'Jingle Bells'. Unfortunately, I was still shaking them in tune to the next carol, the sombre 'In the Bleak Midwinter' and The Teenager was mortified.

On Boxing Day, I went out early for the newspapers and had to pick up some wine for a party later on. Believe me, it's very embarrassing paying for two bottles of wine at 8am when everyone behind me in the queue is buying satsumas and milk. Especially when my hands are playing up again and the wine bottles rattled in my bag as if I was having tremors from alcohol withdrawal.

Anyway, MS-wise, I've been more tired than usual and have spent endless hours lolling around on the sofa, wrapped in a duvet. My feet have been buzzing more and the foot drop is driving me mad. I also had a spectacular argument with my bookcase. The bookcase won and my upper arm is covered in a violent purple bruise and throbs incessantly.

Apart from that, I'm looking forward to more days of too much of everything. I have two very large boxes of chocolates that I feel deserve my undivided attention and a bag of Twiglets in the cupboard, just in case. What more could I possibly need?

31st December 2012

The Last Day of The Year

So, here we are, the very last day of the year and what a year it's been. I've been diagnosed with MS, had Alemtuzumab treatment, lost my job and started a new one. As one door closes, another one opens and all that. A whole fresh new year is ready to be discovered. Exciting!

So why oh why are two of the most miserable songs *ever* written all about New Year? Honestly, if I hear 'Happy New Year' by Abba one more time, I'll be in danger of becoming seriously depressed and full of Nordic noir-ishness. And I'm dreading U2's 'New Years Day' playing on an endless loop all day Tuesday. Where's the happiness? Where's the looking forward to a bright, shiny new year?

A random sample of Abba's 'Happy New Year' lyrics include:

- Here we are, me and you, feeling lost and feeling blue
- It's the end of the party, and the morning seems so grey
- Seems to me now, that the dreams we had before are all dead,
- nothing more

Makes you want to crack open the champagne and fire off some party poppers, eh?

I guess New Year's Eve *can* be a bit depressing - we look over the past year, sigh over some of our decisions and ponder our regrets.

According to the newspapers, most of us will be at home, celebrating with a Marks and Spencer's £10 meal deal. We'll count down to Big Ben and toast the New Year in with a shrug of the shoulders and head for bed at 12.10am.

But this year, I want to celebrate my achievements and the fact that I survived everything life and MS had to throw at me. I'm still here! And I'm stronger and happier than I have been in a long time. The MS community has embraced me and I have found incredible support from other MSers. My family and friends have been amazing. What's not to like? So, sorry Abba. I won't be singing along to your dirge today. I will be having a nice glass of wine, chilling in a wine bar with jazz playing in the background. Goodbye 2012, I'm sure 2013 will be one of my best years yet.

2nd January 2013

Back To Life, Back To Reality

Christmas and New Year are well and truly over and it's back to work today. I am torn. Part of me is excited and full of plans for the year ahead, yet part of me will miss the lovely unreality of the last few weeks.

After a truly terrible year, it was a chance to kick back, relax and recover. Aside from celebrating Christmas, catching up with friends and family and all the usual over-indulgence, Christmas is an excellent excuse for suspending real life. Normal routine is put on hold and I could say, 'Oh, I'll do that next year'.

Well, now it *is* next year and reality is breathing down my neck. Even though I worked between Christmas and New Year, it felt different, as there were still ongoing celebrations to look forward to. Christmas time cushioned me in magical possibilities. Dreams can come true and weird and wonderful plans were discussed late into the night, the Christmas lights twinkling softly in the background.

I will be taking them down in the next day or so and will miss them and all my lovely decorations. Oh, and the chocolate coins and Christmas cake. I will miss the sense of expectation in the air. Stripped of the Christmas trappings, life comes back into sharp focus once more.

Anyway, I guess it's time to concentrate on the here and now. The Teenager comes back from London on Saturday and normal routine will definitely be back with a rude bang - the schoolwork, the laundry, the rugby matches, the grunts, the mysteriously-vanishing food.

My final year at University starts in February and I will once more be knee-deep in study notes, essays and books. Does anyone else find January a dreary and grey month? The only thing to look forward to is Valentine's Day. If you have a partner. Which I don't.

I was joking with a friend the other day about how hard it would be to find a new man in my situation. If it was tricky enough before being diagnosed with MS - 30-something, divorced, single mother. Imagine my lonely hearts advert now: 30-something, divorced, single mother and oh, by the way I have MS. I mean, what are the chances?

11th January 2013

Why 'Stumbling In Flats?'

I've had some messages asking me to explain the title of my blog, so get yourselves comfortable and I will tell you the whole sorry saga.

I'm quite tall for a woman, and I was pretty tall in school. I longed to be a dinky little thing, one of those cute girls the rugby blokes would be quick to take under their wing and look after. No such luck. So, I slouched. I wore Doc Martin boots, long skirts edged with tiny mirrors and grungy tops.

All through sixth form, I was group-less, so belonged to the group of all the people who didn't belong to any group. When I was 18, I decided against taking up my place in University and moved to Europe instead. I swapped the grunge for crisp white shirts and smart jeans, and if I was feeling particularly adventurous, a jaunty neck-scarf.

The next step was exchanging my Doc Martins for elegant, Italian-made leather ankle boots, with a glorious heel. Well, it was a life-changer. I did not walk, I strode. I sashayed. Head and shoulders back, I adored strutting my stuff.

I had a bit of a setback in Poland though, when a bunch of friends and I headed off to stock up on cheap fags and beer. We ended up staying in a dodgy hostel where we were told to leave our shoes outside the door. Polish tradition, no?

The next morning, my beautiful boots were gone. I cried. A lot. I drove back home in a borrowed pair of too-small flip-flops. Lesson learned, I saved up for another pair and never looked back. Until MS came along.

I may as well have been walking on stilts. I simply could no longer wear heels at all. My 'walk' became a ridiculous shuffle, eyes downcast, watching the floor. Foot drop was the bane of my life.

So, with a heavy heart, I gave my last two pairs of heels to a good friend of mine. It was a sad, sad day. And since then, the closest I have to heels are cowboy boots. How depressing. I miss my walk. I miss striding. I hate foot drop. But it's happened. I have a whole bunch of beautiful flat shoes. But, hey, I still stumble.

8

Barbara A Stensland

12ᵗʰ January 2013

Bring On The Snow

We are overjoyed in our little household that there may
be snow on the way. The Teenager is happy because it
could mean a day or two off school. I'm obviously not
happy about that, but I love snow.

Apart from it looking pretty, I love it because it makes
some of MS's horrible side-effects socially acceptable.
Honestly! Let me explain.

I have foot drop. Some days it doesn't happen (but
you're always waiting for it to) and some days it's constant.
Wandering around the shops is not always an attractive
option, It's more a case of smash and grab a few groceries
and head home. But if it snows, we all belong to The
Ministry of Silly Walks.

Foot drop is hidden when you're trudging through
snow. Everyone is watching where they put their feet, not
just me. It's lovely. And if I fall over, well, lots of people
do in the snow, and at least there should be a soft landing.

I also like the suspension of real life and the feeling that
we're in the grip of a National Crisis. We start to look out
for our neighbours, whoever gets to the shops first buys
milk for everyone and we smile as we walk/stumble past
other people in the street. I used to live in a country where
it snowed for over half the year. Everyone was pretty blasé

98

about it but I was like a kid at Christmas, 'ooooh it's snowing, look!' 'Yes, dear, it does that a lot here.'

Snow wasn't very kind to me back then though. I skidded in my car and landed upside down at the side of the road in the middle of nowhere. I clambered out and walked home, crying all the way. I wasn't hurt, just stunned that snow could be so mean.

Then there was the time I was convinced I'd make a great skier. How hard could it be? Answer - very difficult when everyone else in that country was born with skis strapped to their feet. On the nursery slope (called nursery for a very, very good reason) toddlers whizzed past me at electrifying speed pausing only to point at the adult inching painfully forwards, legs akimbo.

I called it a day and never went back. Anyway, I'm watching all the weather forecasts, as is The Teenager. We're keeping our fingers crossed.

15th January 2013

Why Work?

Quite soon after my MS diagnosis, a few people asked me when I would be giving up work. I was stunned. Surely now, more than ever, I would need the security of a routine, wages and the confidence boost a rewarding job can give?

It seemed to me that to stop work was an old-fashioned view and had no place in the 21st century, when there was so much understanding and support in place (my last workplace a huge exception). I now stand corrected. Recent research uncovered the depressing facts:

- More than 75% of people with MS report that the condition has affected their employment and career opportunities.

- Up to 80% of people with MS stop working within 15 years of the onset of the condition.

- Up to 44% of people with MS retire early because of their condition.

- People with MS lose an average of 18 working years.

The report states that with the right support, people with MS could continue to live full and productive lives for much longer, yet during periods of economic downturn and job losses, people with long term health problems feel especially vulnerable.

Research shows that many employers lack knowledge about the condition and may not always understand that the needs of employees with MS can and should be accommodated in the workplace. MS is often a 'hidden disease' and the extent of its impact is not visible to others and over 80% of us are affected by fatigue.

In my case, my chosen career path has veered off in a completely different direction than pre-MS. I was steadily building towards a new career once The Teenager was old enough for me to work full-time. I am a matter of months away from completing my second degree.

It's ironic. Just when my whole life was opening up, when I could put the years of child-care behind me and finally take on a much fuller role in my career, along comes MS and puts paid to my plans. Life has a funny way of turning round and smacking us in the face when we least expect it.

I could either crumple or make the best of a whole new situation and right now, I'm planning to work for as long as I possibly can.

18ᵗʰ January 2013

Snow Joke

It's finally here. The white stuff is falling from the sky and there's a *lot* of it. The Teenager is flapping around trying to find his gloves so he can make snowballs and I doubt school will be open today.

Last week, when the promised snow failed to materialise, he was nonchalant. 'Don't care. Too old for snowballs anyway. D'uh. Snow's for kids.' Hmm. That's why he rushed to the window every morning and turned away each time with a sad little face.

The news is on and this is now obviously a National Crisis. Who would've thought it - snow in winter? They have cold-looking reporters in padded jackets stationed across the country, sending live and 'exclusive' reports from gritting depots, fields of snow and um, gritting depots.

My friend texted me yesterday, saying people were panic-buying petrol, there was no bread or milk left in the supermarket and the roads were jammed. Guess we'll be having Pot Noodles and biscuits for lunch then.

This is pretty bad timing for me though. I was all booked in with the MS rapid access clinic due to some eye problems, but it was cancelled an hour later due to the forecast snow. So I will use the time to try out my Nordic walking poles. I've already got my wellies ready and a backpack to put my shopping in.

I'm going to look ridiculously stupid, but no one cares in the snow. Hopefully. Luckily, I am not back in work until next week so I'm going to spend this time sorting out my university books and look over my notes to remind myself how to write an impressive essay. It's been a while.

I have a pot full of brand new pens and highlighters, the printer is full of ink and I even have little sticky notes in four different colours to mark interesting and informative points in my books. All I need now is for my rusty brain to click in to gear and I'll be fine.

So, I'm off to dig out the thermals, check the ski poles and head off to the shops as soon as I'm ready. I may be some time....

19th January 2013

Not Such a Clever Idea

Ok, who suggested I should take some ski poles and go out walking in the white stuff?

And it all started so well. At 7am yesterday morning I was doing a little stumbly jig in the snow outside my house, the cat glaring at me from the window. Gloves, hooded jacket and ski poles were primed and ready to go, so I had a bit of a quick trial run, eventually deciding I looked less like a weirdo with just the one.

The Teenager was busy messaging his friends while I got myself loaded up. Keys? Check. Mobile? Check. Wallet? Check. Huge ruck-sack? Check. Emergency ration biscuits? Check.

I headed off, feeling a bit silly with the solitary ski pole, especially when someone yelled, 'oi, you lost one!' at me from the other side of the road. So far, so good though. I trekked up to the shops, feeling intrepid and adventurous and soon got into a semi-comfortable stride. Any foot drop I had was hidden by the snow.

I got to the supermarket, but snowpocalypse had already struck. There was no bread, no potatoes, not much meat and hardly any fruit left. The shelves had been stripped bare.

I picked up some grotty mushrooms, half-price bacon, Monster Munch crisps and a tub of double cream (no idea why, seemed a good idea). After a quick coffee pit-stop, I trekked up the hill to my mum's with a newspaper, another coffee, then over to Tom, the elderly guy I check in on. Stopped for a tea and a chat, then trekked back up to the shops to meet a friend for coffee, eventually getting home four hours after I set off.

My cheeks were ablaze, I felt exhilarated and generally rather fab. Until I took my welly boots off and collapsed in a heap in the hall. Excruciating cramp in my legs, a sore hand from gripping my ski pole and a huge wave of tiredness sent me straight to my sofa. My legs and feet are still tingling and buzzing.

Think I got a bit carried away.

23rd January 2013

That Annoys You? Oh Really?

I was quite happily waiting at the doctor's surgery for my monthly blood test yesterday, when I picked up a newspaper. There was a full-page article devoted to things that 'make women seethe.' Interest piqued, I read further, expecting to see examples such as schools still closed since last week, the shocking price of petrol or the lies men tell on dating websites (and the 10-year-old photos they post up).

Well. Oh, to have a life where stepping on Lego or forgetting to turn the dishwasher on was all that made me curse. Apparently, the following everyday annoyances can make a woman rage:

- Misjudging kettle water levels

- Getting an itchy nose while washing up

- Useless ribbon loops sewn into clothes

- When the wind blows your hair into your lip gloss

- Getting a full bag out of a pedal bin

- Catching your sleeve on a door handle

Well, excuse me if I don't rush over with tea and sympathy. I also object to the misogynistic tone of the article, which places women fully in the 'helpless, silly people' category, where all we worry about is putting too much water in the kettle or how to deal with tangled wire coat hangers.

Let's leave the serious issues to the men, don't worry your pretty little head, there's a good girl, eh? This may as well be journalism from the 1950s. Can you imagine a similar article, yet written about men? Would men really rage about scratchy clothes labels, a tissue in the wash or needing to drain a 'no drain' tuna can? Anyway, in the interest of balance, here's my MS list of everyday things that make me seethe:

- People thinking I'm drunk after half a glass of wine

- My robot, wonky walk when my legs won't work properly

- Waking up half-blind

- Tripping over my own feet. Repeatedly.

- Reaching for my coffee cup and knocking it over

- Not being able to wear heels

- Trying to explain fatigue for the zillionth time

I'd better stop there. I could go on. And on. But I just got lemon juice in my eye and I am seriously raging.....

24th January 2013

Fun In The Bathroom

The snowpocalypse has meant I have spent an awful lot of time at home, which has given me an awful lot of time to stare at the mould creeping along my bathroom walls. Finally, I have had enough.

In the old days, pre-MS, I could paint the bathroom in half a day, whizzing around barely stopping for breath. This time, I will need to approach the project with caution, precision and a battle plan. So the other day, I began.

After trudging up to the doctor's for my blood test, I trudged back to the paint shop. I had done my research. I knew I needed an anti-mould solution, an interior seal damp and, finally, paint, so I asked the guy for help finding them. 'But why do you need all that stuff?' he asked. Well, the bathroom is exploding with mould, it's horrible. 'It can't be that bad, surely, how old is your house?'

Oh dear. Obviously women shouldn't know anything about painting or preparing surfaces, yada yada yada. I gave him my best steely look, gritted my teeth and informed him the house is 160 years old, the window sills are over a foot thick and if the damp has gone in that far, I've got a serious problem.

He gave in, but got the last laugh, thrusting a couple of paint brochures into my hand before I left, saying 'here,

take these, they've got some lovely pretty colours in there.'
I stomped home in mood.

I don't care if I paint the bathroom in 'ocean ripple',
'chic shadow' or 'urban obsession', as long as it gets done.
If I had my way, I'd paint it all black so I'd never have to
see the mould again.

Anyway, I am all set to go, but nothing has been done.
Three reasons: my arms get tingly and numb if I hold them
up for too long, my balance won't be the best on step-
ladders and I worry about suddenly get tired half-way
through. The guy in the shop didn't quite succeed in
making me feel completely stupid and girly, but MS
certainly has.

26th January 2013

Are We Our Own Worst Enemies?

Are MSers guilty of naval-gazing and deconstructing every single little symptom and therefore preventing ourselves from being understood by other people? And I'll start with the term 'MSer'.

There has been a huge amount of debate in the MS forums and on Twitter about whether it is 'acceptable' to call ourselves MSers. I mean, really. If we are pitting ourselves against each other in this matter, what hope is there for us?

I use the term a lot. I think it's snappy, short and easy for social media. Whether or not you choose to 'define' yourself as a MSer is up to you, but don't berate those who do. I may refer to myself a MSer, but I certainly don't live my life solely as a person with MS. It just happens to be part of my life, the same as being a mother, a daughter, a sister, a colleague, etc.

Once you're diagnosed with MS, ok, you join a whole load of other people with MS, but we are all different, just as daughters, mothers and sisters are - they generally only have that one thing in common. And yes, MSers can be incredibly guilty of dissecting and discussing each tiny symptom, blowing things out of proportion. Wait - before I get hate mail - I have been there (still am sometimes). I hold my hand up.

Pre-diagnosis, I was a frequent visitor on MS forums. I was scared, bewildered, anxious and lacking in information, and often the forums made me more worried, not less. I started this blog to show the funny, embarrassing and downright socially awkward side of MS, precisely because I was so fed up reading blogs and forums that were simply a litany of endless complaints. Who wants to read about that? If we want sympathy and understanding from other people, constant moaning is not the way to go about it.

I know some of my posts are downbeat, but I hope the majority can raise a smile and an 'oh, that happens to me too!' We need to amaze people - 'THIS is what MS looks like' - 'Hey, I'm still living, working, laughing, being happy'. Reach down to those going through the diagnostic process, befriend them and inspire them. Maybe then we can stop this cycle of despair.

30th January 2013

Muddy Hell

The Teenager had a rugby match on Sunday. After the snow thawed, the torrential rain came so we were convinced the match would be cancelled. A pitch inspection was due the day before and after the groundsman had waded through inches of mud he declared the pitch good to play. Of course.

The Teenager had a lift with the trainer and off he went with his Lucozade and boot bag. Three hours later he was returned, a huge blob of mud standing on the doorstep. The only un-muddy bit of him was a grubby bandage wound tightly round his wrist, which he held out pitifully with a pained expression.

He'd only played for ten minutes (so who knows how much more mud he could have gathered if he'd played full time), as someone had trod on his wrist during a try and he was out for the rest of the game.

Anyway, he stripped, I picked up the sodden clothes and chucked them in the machine as he squelched his way to the shower.

Within ten minutes, there was a yell: 'Muuuuuuuuuuuuum!' 'What?' 'I'm in aaaaagony. But we won, 43-0.' 'Glad you won! Ok, I'll bandage it up, don't worry. Then you can go and do some homework.' 'Too sore. I'm dying'. 'Ok, just do it quietly'.

Believe me, I *was* sympathetic, but this continued in a loop all day. He'd appear in front of me, a wan-faced vision. He'd lie on the sofa, asking for help to pick up the remote, but oddly not needing the same help to play on his iPhone.

I made him a hot chocolate with a dollop of Fluff on top and helped him pack his school bag for Monday. I bandaged, unbandaged and bandaged his wrist so many times I lost count. It got in the way of his x-box controller. I got a bigger bandage (ha!) and wrapped that round his wrist instead.

I'm not a horrible mum, honestly, but my nerves were stretched. One sulky Teenager plus one (very slight) injury has made for a very unhappy household these last few days.

To top it all, after helping him with his school jumper yesterday morning and packing his school bag once more, I offered to bandage his wrist again. 'Nah, don't worry, it felt better on Monday, I just enjoyed wearing it, everyone was asking me about it at school......'

5th February 2013

Arthouse Bingo

The Teenager was away at the weekend, so I went to an arty café/wine bar/arts space to pretend to be cultivated, arty and interesting.

Hopefully my pale, MS-tired face added to the mystique. To pass the time and look as if I am writing an angsty novel, I play 'Arthouse Bingo'.

The rules are easy - a point if you can spot each of the following, and if you get to 5, buy yourself another drink:

- Massively over-sized lampshades, preferably in black.

- No menus, just a huge blackboard with locally-sourced food, i.e. they went to the local Lidl, bought some salami and Parma ham and slapped it on a slate tile with a couple of sliced gherkins.

- A higher than average array of beardy men (and some women). Likewise, a higher than average amount of red trousers worn.

- A minimum of 30 European beers with 'ironic' names - the easy way to get intellectually inebriated.

- Lots of conversations starting with, 'But is it art?'

- A tribe of wild-looking children running amok as the parents look on indulgently, 'Juniper, Hugo and Mabel, darlings, untie Milly and come and eat your asparagus soldiers.'

- A book-swap corner - a bookcase where you can bring your old tat and swap it for a 1992 Driving Atlas of France.

- Coffee must be handpicked by an organic wizard in deepest Columbia.

- Lots of women with flowing hair, strings of hand-made beads and jangly silver bracelets.

- Old Skool puddings on the menu - spotted dick, apple crumble, custard, etc. Such fun!

- At least 5 terribly anguished-looking people hunched over MacBooks.

- If there is a cinema, listen out for, 'Oh, but I preferred the book, the original Dutch translation.'

- Everyone speaks very LOUDLY. No need for music unless there is a visiting harmonica group from Patagonia.

Anyway, I passed a lovely couple of hours, braying loudly, speculating as to whether the huge painting in the bar was art or not. I rattled my beads intelligently and enjoyed my ironic glass of dry white wine.

I have past form in these places - as a teenager, I considered myself to be the coolest person ever, standing by the bar, beret on, reading Jean-Paul Sartre and talking utter nonsense.

If I had the nerve (and legs), I would love to turn up in a denim mini-skirt and white stilettos. Only two flaws with that plan - one, I can't walk in heels and two, the crowd would probably think I was the performance art.

7th February 2013

Skydiving or an Adjustable Bed?

I love MS magazines. It's important to keep up to date with latest developments, policy and research. That to one side, I'm confused.

On the one hand, there are articles about 'triumph over adversity' - people with MS skydiving, firewalking, trekking the world despite all the odds. On the other, the adverts paint a very different picture - catheters, adjustable beds, respite care, Motability, bath lifts, etc. So which is it to be?

Which camp do I fall into? Well, neither. I'm not brave enough to triumph over my adversity. The nearest I got to skydiving was when my friend jumped out of a tiny plane over the Arizona desert on his 40th. I was so traumatised to see him suddenly drop out of a plane that I clung to the bemused pilot until we landed.

I'm also, thankfully, not at the stage yet where I need to consider a versatile, easy access shower or electric scooter. I know many of us are, don't get me wrong, but where is the middle ground? I feel both inadequate and scared. Are these the only two ways to live with MS?

I'm probably a typical person with MS - in my 30's, with a child, trying to hold down a job and worrying about things we all worry about, MS or not; the bills, the economy, hoodies, the NHS, the price of food. I haven't got the time, or childcare, to set off for China or raise thousands and thousands of pounds.

I do what I can to support MS charities. I trained as a support volunteer. I'm in a working group. I attend meetings and rallies ('I'm not a scrounger, I have MS'). In my own little way, I hope my blog too, can show that life goes on with MS. I used to work in advertising, I know companies are particular about where they place their ads. So why do they ignore us?

There's 100,000 of us in the UK alone. I want to see adverts for restaurants, travel companies (not just insurance), sparkly flat shoes, make-up, days out. I will jump (carefully) off my soap-box now. Rant over. Is it just me?

8th February 2013

Off My Trolley

Since MS turned my brain to mush, supermarkets confuse me, trip me up and make me buy things I don't want (travel toothbrush, pom-pom air freshener for the car). I've successfully managed to avoid them for the last month or so, but the list of things I couldn't buy locally got longer and longer and I finally had to take the plunge.

Yesterday was the big day. I made a cafetiere of coffee, strong and black, for courage. I gathered my shopping bags together, got my list, double-checked it. I could do this. I was ready. Drove off.

Turned round. Forgot my wallet. Drove off. Got parked. Checked lippy in mirror and I was good to go. Wrestled with trolley and yanked it into the store. Deep breath.

Huh? They've changed the layout round *again*? Now I had to go up and down every single aisle. The Teenager needed ingredients for a baking lesson in school. He told me he needs a huge jar of Nutella (I was born yesterday) and the cat wanted to try a different brand of food.

I picked up the bin bags, the envelopes, the printer paper, the cat food, the garlic, the shoe polish. Excellent. Just about got everything on the list and avoided the end-of-aisle offers. Only the Nutella to go. The place was lovely and quiet and I glided around feeling serene and calm.

My final aisle. I swerve past a parked trolley when I hear, 'What are YOU doing here? We thought you were ill, but you look so well?'. Oh god. It's that mother from school. The one with the most intelligent child in the universe.

I listened to her reel off the prodigy's most recent accomplishments, made my excuses and left, zooming (wonkily) straight for the checkout. Got to the car. Fabulous. The car next to me was parked so close, I couldn't open the driver's door.

I stomped around, then stomped around some more. With a dramatic sigh, I flung myself into the passenger seat then very inelegantly shifted myself over into the driver's seat with a lot of huffing and puffing.

Drove home, chucked a meal in the microwave and sighed. Then I got a pen and piece of paper and started my new list. Can't wait for next month.

9th February 2013

A Helping Hand in Limboland

Sometimes I wish I could go back in time to that terrifying morning when I woke up and couldn't speak properly or walk in a straight line. If I knew then what I know now, I would have been a very different person.

For someone whose father had MS, I knew surprisingly little. I had no idea what CIS was, what an MRI would show, why I had to have a lumbar puncture. I was in Limboland. I might develop MS. Or I might not. It is a cruel waiting game.

I didn't understand the 'multiple' part of multiple sclerosis. I left the clinic after that first relapse utterly petrified. What was I to do now? I had been given a couple of MS leaflets and information about how to contact the MS team. But if I didn't yet have MS, why would I be given that? I was bewildered.

I accessed a few forums, one dedicated to Limbolanders and I gained a huge amount of information; the forums were a lifeline, but at a cost.

A lot of people had been stuck in Limboland for years, some well over a decade. Despair and anger oozed from the forum. We were all in a nasty, dark waiting room and I would feel a painful stab of strange envy when someone posted that they had been diagnosed, and were now leaving us behind; they had the golden ticket.

I read everything I could about the McDonald criteria, ticking off the four points bit by bit. Finally (but only 10 months later), I had my ticket. My brain threw up more lesions, far too many and I was diagnosed. Possibly one of the best and worst days of my life.

I wish I had been handed a step-by-step guide to life in Limboland, clearly explaining the whole diagnostic process, the frustrations, the waiting. Could someone please publish this? Letting us know that you have to go through so much, from first relapse to eventual diagnosis.

Break us in gently. Please don't throw us in the deep end. So, to everyone diagnosed with MS, look out for the Limbolanders. Treat them kindly. Be an inspiration and show them we are not so bad, it's not so scary. There is a life after diagnosis. Aren't we all proof of this?

11th February 2013

The Plugholes Are Now Sparkling

I have also done three loads of laundry, washed all the cushion covers, baked a banana and walnut loaf, cleaned the fridge, shredded a huge pile of paperwork and sorted out my kitchen cupboards. Domestic diva? I wish.

It appears I would rather pluck a bunch of yucky hairs from the plugholes with a wooden barbecue skewer than sit down and study. I have one year left of a six-year part time degree course. I could have graduated last year, without honours, but I'm awkward like that. Or a masochist.

University officially started on Saturday, but I didn't. I tried. I laid out all the books, printed off loads of information, stocked up on post-it notes, new pens, a brand new folder. I sit at my desk, scrolling through the online learning guides, thinking, 'oh, how interesting' for about 15 seconds, then click over to my Twitter feed instead.

Yesterday I sat down to read the newspaper for five minutes and an hour later I had read it from cover to cover. Who knew the letters page and obituaries could be so fascinating? I can blame MS for this, but only partly.

At the end of the last academic year I was in the middle of a pretty major relapse, the steroids were keeping me up all night and my brain was in meltdown. It refused to remember one single fact, one theory. I struggled through and gleefully chucked the notes in the bin after the exam last July.

Now, 7 months later, it's hard to pick up the thread again. The thought of planning and writing an essay fills me with dread. Researching, indexing, referencing all seem like scientific impossibilities. I have printed off our official Harvard reference guide (all 35 pages of it) and have only read up to page 8.

To prove I could do it, I pulled out all my essays from last year. Bad move. Who wrote these? They were pretty good and I was impressed until I realised I had written them. My standards were obviously a lot higher back then.

I will muddle through. I will play with the post-it notes and highlight noteworthy points in my books. I'm hoping that if I read the same pages over and over again I will absorb the facts by osmosis. Until then, I have the vacuum cleaner filter to wash and lightbulbs to polish.

13th February 2013

I Stumble, Therefore I Am

I caught the tail-end of a programme the other day in which a man with a prosthetic foot was being interviewed. He was asked if, should a miracle cure become available, would he take it? He was vociferous in his rejection of this - he was perfectly happy and his 'disability' had made him who he was.

Powerful stuff. Mulling it over, I came to a surprising conclusion. MS has shaped and moulded me in completely unexpected and positive ways and given me courage where previously I had very little.

When I was younger I was in a terrible, near-fatal car crash. I vowed to change my life forever if I recovered, and I would never take anything for granted again. A year later, the scars had almost healed, I could walk properly and I was back to normal. Did I carry that message and always remember how fragile life was? Did I heck.

But with something like MS, there is no end point, no point at which you can forget, so we really do need to change our lives and keep changing them, whilst appreciating every small victory and achievement.

I used to hate MS, until I realised that by hating it, I was hating a fundamental part of myself and this was essentially self-loathing. MS is me and I am MS. It is not a separate entity. I went through a dark, lonely, terrifying grieving process and hit rock bottom not just once but repeatedly.

When a chink of light appeared, I was on the up again. I frequently think that when you get diagnosed with MS, anything else is immaterial. You can cope with pretty much everything life has to throw at you. And I think that is true and a powerful lesson to learn at my age, rather than as a wistful pensioner looking back over a life less-lived.

MS has given me a kick up the backside. It has made me speak up for myself, it has made me more confident and less willing to accept shabby behaviour. My stumbling, my tingling, and dodgy hands are now part of me. I stumble, therefore I am.

14th February 2013

Flowers, Who Needs 'Em?

Yes, I am a singleton on Shameless Commercialism Day. Valentine's Day. But the good news is, at least I'm not working in an office any more. Long gone are those awful days when everyone else received bouquets of flowers, accompanied by 'oh, I didn't know that was going to happen' squeals from various women jumping up and down at the sight of a few roses.

The same women who, a week earlier, could be heard saying in the toilets, '...I've told him, if he doesn't send me flowers this year, he can whistle for, you know...' Now my inadequacy is shared only with the cat (she watches the letterbox every day) and she's on my side.

I whinge to friends that I hate the tacky commercialism of Valentine's Day and my heart sinks when all the gooey stuff appears in the shops on Boxing Day. No sooner have the 'Merry Christmas, my squidgy, squashy Boyfriend' cards been packed away, I'm assaulted by a sea of red and pink. And roses. And fluffy little teddy bears with 'I Wuv You' scrawled across their chests.

And what's this whole thing with chocolates? Oi, loved-up people, you get the flowers, you get the meal out, you get the jewellery. Can't you keep your smug little paws off the chocolate - it's for us single ladies. See it as our consolation prize.

Of course, if I was loved-up, I would be starry-eyed with rapture at being presented with a dozen red roses, a Tiffany necklace and a huge box of pralines (my favourites). I would benevolently smile down upon the lesser, single mortals, with pity and not a little smugness. May they too find love, poor, sad, lonely peeps.

But I'm not loved-up, so I can't. Sniff. This Valentine's Day then, I will mostly be listening to 'I Am Woman' (over and over again), hoovering up the Maltesers I stashed away from The Teenager and sitting on the sofa in my comfiest, slobbiest pyjamas. I may even put a face pack on and paint my toenails. Valentine's Day? Meh.

18th February 2013

Putting On Mascara With Boxing Gloves

Ever tried putting mascara on wearing boxing gloves? Or holding a lovely cup of hot coffee? Pretty tough.

My last relapse affected my hands and just for a laugh, they still play up every so often and this weekend was no exception. Like most relapses, it came out of the blue. One day I was elegant(ish) and my hands were just things that did things hands normally do. I didn't really give them much thought.

Until the morning I flicked the kettle on and knocked it over, swiftly followed by my cup. Odd. When I left the house that morning, I missed the door handle. Odder.

I tried to explain to the MS nurse that my hands were either a few seconds too quick or a few seconds too slow, they drop things unexpectedly and sometimes they're so numb, they feel like boxing gloves. It doesn't sound like such a huge problem, but socially it's dire. Putting on make-up is comical - I gave up on eyeliner months ago and mascara wands hurt like hell when they're poked in the eyes.

Lipstick goes on well until, blam, whoops, dodgy line - The Rocky Horror Show's got nothing on me. Wine glasses are a minefield. I've smashed countless. Be warned, never clink glasses with me, just say cheers and nod. All my plates and bowls are chipped and you can hear me doing the washing up a mile away.

If I'm walking through a cutesy, arty gift shop, I have to keep my hands rigidly by my side or ever so carefully reach out, inch by inch, to pick something up. I can clear a shelf of pottery in one fell swoop. And my days of playing KerPlunk and Operation are long gone.

I used to like craft work but can't knit anymore and the glue gun's been in the drawer so long it's seized up. I tried to make a Christmas wreath out of paper hearts and glued everything except the paper. The cat made herself scarce so now I scroll through Pinterest and sigh wistfully.

I persevere though. I am going to invest in melamine plates and plastic wine glasses and I will make that wreath by next Christmas if it kills me. If you see it, be polite and please don't snigger.

21st February 2013

Hospital Bed Booked

I had a letter a couple of days ago confirming that I've been booked in to hospital for my follow-up Alemtuzumab treatment in July. Last year I was in for five days and four nights. This year, only three days and two nights.

Looking back on it, I was a complete hospital novice. So here's my list of what I will be doing differently this time around:

> • Pack my own pillows. The hospital ones (if you are lucky enough to get one) are super-thin slices of foam. And that's being generous.

> • I won't be taking a huge pile of books. I ended up reading only newspapers and trashy magazines, but I did learn a lot about Heidi and Spencer Pratt's marriage and Cheryl Cole's beauty routine.

> • Staying overnight in a Neuro Day Unit means you have absolutely no privacy all day. People come and go for tests and treatments, usually bringing a bunch of family members with them. It's like having a whole load of strangers parading through your bedroom. Must also remember to lie when people ask me if lumbar punctures hurt (they do, I was a screaming banshee).

• Cannulas hurt like hell too and it has to stay in the whole time. Must get it strapped up when not in use as do not want to recreate the Psycho shower scene like last year.

• Much as I loved the regular tea trolley trundling around at all hours, it tastes awful. Will make regular trips downstairs for the hard stuff.

• Accept all the sleeping tablets I can get my hands on - hospital beds are uncomfortable, some lights stay on all night and there are strange people wailing down the corridor.

I will be a calm, confident patient. I know the score this time round. Still a sobering experience though, when the reality of MS really kicks in, far more than just putting up with symptoms on a day to day basis. This is real. The doctor says so.

So when everyone else is packing for a week in the sun, spare a thought for me as I pack my pyjamas, fluffy slippers and selection of snacks to munch on (Jelly Babies, dried banana slices and cookies).

God knows what I'll look like walking through the hospital corridors on my way to book in, struggling with a huge bag and two pillows under my arm. One other point - do hospitals have wi-fi? How will I stay up to date with my blog and Twitter?

23rd February 2013

Sick or What?

Adapting to the role of a sick person is not easy. Society makes it very clear - if you are ill, you must want to get better and you must co-operate with the medical establishment. In return, society will 'allow' you to shed normal responsibilities of work and household tasks for a limited time, until you are better. You are recognised as being in need of care and unable to get better by yourself.

This theory was first developed by Talcott Parsons in 1951 and, despite its shortcomings, still holds firm in most people's minds. But what happens if you have MS, your illness fluctuates and often you are well enough to participate fully in society? Where do you stand then?

MS can mark you out as a fraud. Some things said to me over the last two years:

- 'But you look so well.'

- 'When are you giving up work?'

- 'Wow, you're drinking alcohol.'

- 'I thought you were ill.'

- 'Why are you so tired, you were fine yesterday?'

Living as a fairly young person, with a fairly invisible illness renders you an uncomfortable anomaly. I have no standard 'markers' of a sick person, no visual clues. People just have to take my word for it, and this is where the tension arises.

I am in a no-man's land between being well and being ill. I still want the 'privileges' that being well and a productive member of society brings - a job, a social life, status, etc. Yet I also need the exemption when I am ill, the extra support and help and many people, and society, would much prefer it if I chose one scenario and stuck to it.

I can either be fully productive and keep quiet, or give in and take up the sick role full time. Other people with MS can be just as judgmental. I once went to an MS support group and felt very out of place and unwelcome. Finally, the organiser took me to one side and gently explained that I made the others uncomfortable.

I was talking about work and going out for a meal that evening. He said that this group meeting was often the only outing they had in two weeks. I wasn't 'sick' enough to join their group. I never went back. What's the solution? I have no idea.....

25th February 2013

Unexpected Item In The Blogging Area

I did it. I finally did it. I have popped my internet grocery shopping cherry. What's the big deal? Well, I have a love/hate relationship with supermarkets - they love me and I hate them.

A fellow blogger, Steve, possibly exasperated by my constant complaining, kindly offered to send me a £20 voucher offer for Ocado (for non-UK'ers - a very posh supermarket - far too posh for me to visit in my builder's gear) and yesterday morning, I bit the bullet. And Scottish people never turn down twenty quid.

I got myself prepared. Large sheet of paper, pot of strong coffee and a Sharpie. Ok, jot down all the heavy stuff - cat food, squash, cat food, beans. Then the things I really need - toothbrushes, fish, yoghurt, mince. I was getting into the swing of it. It was time to sign up, log in and go wild in the virtual aisles.

My last attempt at supermarket shopping online was disastrous. I got lost. Then I lost my basket and finally I was off my trolley and I fled, demoralised, bruised and battered by the whole experience. This time round, it was a doddle. I got so carried away, my total had reached over £100 within ten minutes and I hadn't even added the washing-up liquid.

I ruthlessly went through my trolley, chucking out the 3-for-2 ice cream, an expensive skin cream, coloured straws (no idea), 2kg of pasta and a new wok. Better. Before heading for the check-out, I had a little look through the half price offers and treated myself to some kitchen towel and baby sweetcorn. Before you can even get to the check-out, they cleverly throw teasing offers at you, but I resisted and I was let through. All paid, delivery slot booked, done and dusted.

It took twenty minutes and I was still in my dressing gown, jittery after my third cup of filter coffee. I feel very grown up and smart. I may never set foot in a supermarket again. Whoever said MS makes you creative was right - there's always a solution to every little niggle. I have now started a list on my fridge and was dashing back and forth all day, Sharpie in hand, adding things ready for my next shop.

I just hope that when the shopping arrives, there are no substitutes. My friend once ordered a punnet of peaches and found she had been given two tins of them in syrup instead. Not quite the same thing.

27th February 2013

It's Official - I'm A Trendsetter

Yes, that's right, the fashion world has finally listened to me - flat shoes are bang on trend for 2013. Totes amazeballs or what? Crack open the Bolly, dahlings!

According to Roberto Cavalli, speaking from his Milan fashion show, flat shoes are 'cool and it's all coming from London.' Well, ok, I may be 150 miles from London but obviously the fashionistas have heard my anguished pleas and are taking up my cause in droves.

I was far too busy to be interviewed exclusively for Vogue, but luckily, the footwear buying manager for Selfridges was quoted as saying, 'It's a revolution...flats are selling out across every price point.'

After MS cruelly robbed me of my high heels and sashaying walk, I have been resigned to stumbling around in flats, head no longer held high. No one was happier than me when ballet flats briefly flooded the high street, but they're not exactly statement shoes, are they?

Over the last couple of years though, I have slowly built up a nice little collection of smart flats and casual flats, with a pair of Converse thrown in for when I want to 'hang' with The Teenager. He may not let me borrow his SuperDry hoodie (trying too hard to be cool), but he's ok with the blue Converse.

Flats to one side, what other heel-less shoes are cool? Sandals? I don't think so. Flip-flops? Have you seen someone with MS trying to walk in flip-flops? Wellies? Er, no. A fellow Tweeter suggested Doc Martin boots and I did try, but they bring back far too many tragic memories of stomping round various teenage haunts, drinking cider and black (do NOT tell The Teenager) and wearing long skirts. The stripy tights I wore with them still haunt me.

This exciting news has therefore reconfirmed our true status - where us MS'ers lead, the fash-pack follows. Of course, they are down-playing my role in this and are suggesting it's all thanks to the Duchess of Cambridge influencing the new fashion trend, but I reckon Kate's read my blog and has kindly championed me, bless her.

So, I am off to put together some stylish outfits, accessorised with an array of dazzling flats. I may even do that fashion-y thing of putting them in boxes and sticking Polaroids of them on the front - how divine!

1st March 2013

I Fought Back...And Won

I was sacked from my job last October for having MS, preceded by a vicious campaign of bullying and harassment which almost drove me over the edge. At the same time, I was struggling to cope with my diagnosis and had also just been through Alemtuzumab treatment in the summer.

The day I was sacked, I went home in shock. I was at my lowest ebb. The drip-drip effect of the bullying had left me sapped of confidence, drained of energy and incapable of any positive thinking. The sacking was the culmination of a truly horrific year. How anyone can bully a person going through a diagnosis of MS is beyond me and the cruelty of it still astounds me. I decided to accept my fate and leave it at that.

But then I got angry, then furious. Was I really just going to walk away? Luckily, I still had one tiny scrap of fight left in me and so began a long legal process.

I am over the moon to report that I have now won my case. The matter is settled and it is time to move on, with my dignity and pride restored.

Bullying at work can be insidious. It is not always immediately obvious. It can start insignificantly and like an abusive partner, can slowly erode your confidence, your judgement and your rational thinking. When the bullying then escalates, you feel too undermined and isolated to fight back. Bullying someone with MS (or any other serious illness) is cowardly.

The bullying may come from a position of strength, from their status in work, but it is only carried out by weak people who take delight in hurting others who are already in pain. I have fought a long, exhausting battle and was close to giving up along the way, such was the hold these people still had over me in my mind. It's only thanks to family, friends, fellow MSers and a fabulous lawyer that I got to this point.

If you are in the same position I was, don't accept it. You are worth more than that. Keep notes of every incident, no matter how small, and of every date. Surround yourself with a strong network and, most importantly, realise that it is not your fault. It's a beautiful feeling to wake up every morning knowing I am no longer bullied. I am a worthy person and I will go on to better things. As they say, success is the best revenge.

3rd March 2013

I'm Harry Styles' Mother

If you want to feel suddenly ancient, do what I did on Friday and go late-night shopping into town right before a One Direction tour date.

The plan was a good one. The Teenager was at a sleepover, my friend was in town and we were going to hit the shops, followed by a drink or two, perhaps a bite to eat. How cosmopolitan and smart I felt as we left the house. Hmm.

Lots of traffic on the way in, got parked, went to the lift. Hordes of tweenagers jumping up and down squealing at each other, comparing glittery eye-shadow and nail varnish. Swarms of them flooding the shops and restaurants, clutching banners 'I'm Mrs Styles', 'Marry ME Harry', 'One Direction - Over Here'.

In an instant, I felt very, very old and very dowdy as I remembered Harry was only 19 (19!!) and was born in 1994, two years after I left high school. I was old enough to be his mother. My friend wanted to buy a new duvet, and as we were standing feeling up different togs and feathers, working our way up and down the row, I felt even older. Duvet shopping. On a Friday night. Where did it all go wrong?

I bought some cards (ooh, they do a lovely selection in John Lewis), vitamins and a new wallet. Exciting.

Prematurely old? We decided to cut our losses and head to the bars. We wandered around, checking each of them out. Too trendy, too dark, too small, too many doormen, too big, too loud, too scary. We were a walking, talking Dr Seuss poem.

I stopped outside one of them in horror. 'Retro Bar - 90's Music'. Since when were the 90's retro? Dispirited, we sat outside a fake Spanish tapas bar, glumly sipping our wine (me) and gin and tonic (him), watching the skinny, mini-skirted women teetering past on high heels, hair sprayed into submission, faces glowing with anticipation. We muttered to each other, 'she must be freeeezing' and 'why don't they put a warm jacket on?'

We finished our drinks and went home. I put the cat out, popped my slippers on and settled down for a nice night in front of the telly, the lyrics of 'Those Were the Days My Friend' running sadly through my mind. I think it's time to shake things up a little.

7th March 2013

Chronically Ill, Terminally Depressing?

The builder popped over to see me after work the other day. I was on my sofa, floored by MS fatigue, snuggled into my duvet, watching trashy t.v.

As soon as he walked in and saw me, he took a step back, a look of dismay on his face, 'God, I feel depressed just seeing you there like that.' If he'd slapped me across the face with a wet fish, it couldn't have hurt more.

I protested, made a joke about it, but it touched a very raw nerve. I don't want to be depressing. I don't want to be that person on the other side of an invisible divide. I saw myself through his eyes and didn't like what I saw. MS has shoved me under ice. I look the same, but I'm trapped, banging on that ice, yelling pointlessly for my friends on the surface to hear me.

I've had to absorb a lot of changes into my life since MS smashed into it like an unwanted gatecrasher at my party. Some of them are huge, but most are small changes I now take for granted - the afternoon naps, the slower pace of walking, the brain mush. To me they are now normal.

But seeing myself from someone else's viewpoint brings me up short. I can see just how much I have changed and I hate it. Before MS, I was always on the go. I travelled the world, had incredible adventures, and I've been strong, independent and vibrant. Looking at myself now, I can see I have I've become a shadow of that.

My house has become my refuge and I spend far too much time in it. It is comforting. No one can see me trip, hold on to the banisters, drop another glass. I feel safe here. I know the builder didn't mean to hurt with his comment. I probably needed to hear it. I want to get my zest for life back.

MS is a hefty ball and chain to drag through life, but at least if I'm facing forward, I can't see it, even though I know it's there. At the moment I am standing outside the party, nose pressed to the window, watching everyone else's lives unfolding. It's about time I joined in again.

9th March 2013

Nice Face, Shame About the Makeup

I sat down to write my list of things I must do,
completely forgetting that I had actually attempted
something for the first time ever last week. Don't laugh. I
went for a make-up consultation.

Yes, I entered the Glossy Hall of Terror and lived to
tell the tale, albeit with a slightly bruised ego. I had done
my research, knew which counter I wanted and marched
with purpose towards it, then stumbled past the perfume-
sprayers, the ladies who lunch and the gaggle of make-up
ladies, in whose über-manicured hands my fate now rested.

At the counter, I nonchalantly pretended to examine
the nail varnish until an assistant (Hi! I'm Carly!) with
thickly-troweled-on make-up, surprised brows and a
blowfish smile wobbled over to me in her 6 inch heels
(jealous, much?). Out came my sorry tale, the heat
intolerance, the cold intolerance, my poor, ravaged
complexion, my battered soul.

She nodded sympathetically, head cocked to one side as
I pretty much flung myself at her feet, begging for help.
'Now, do you want the 'no-make up, make up look, just
like I'm wearing?' 'Oh, um' (a quick glance at her face
confirming my worst suspicions) 'Well, I was hoping to,
er.....'

'Don't you worry pet, my auntie had cancer, awful it was, so I know just what you're looking for. You want something to help you fight back, face the world, feel strong and feminine again!' 'Well, honestly, I'm just looking to, um, freshen things up a little.'

'Super duper. Now, here's our colours, our brushes, our pots, our testers, our dvd, our loyalty card, our massively overpriced eye cream. And what we do, what's really special, is that I will call you next week, see how you're getting on with your new make-up. Isn't that lovely? A nice little phone call. Should cheer you right up!'

Desperate to leave, I selected the make-up I wanted, chucked in a moisturiser and a primer and wangled some microscopic free samples, then diligently wrote down my telephone number and fled. It was nice and girly to do something different, and some compensation for having such a limited range of shoes to choose from.

Sadly, I still haven't got the hang of blusher quite yet - less English Rose and more Spanish Beach Holiday Mahogany. And I'm still waiting for that special phone call from Carly...

11th March 2013

This Is A Boring Post

'I'm bored. Bored, bored, bored.' (stamps foot) Think this is The Teenager expecting me to entertain him? Nope. It's me talking to a friend.

Something all the leaflets about all the symptoms of MS don't cover is the sheer, mind-numbing boredom that comes with it. MS itself is never boring - there's the unexpected delight of waking up in the morning wondering just what symptom it will chuck at you today, and MS has a whole bag of them. But with these symptoms comes the crushing boredom.

Top of the list is the boredom that comes with having to sleep. A lot. It's a huge time-waster, it's not fun or cushy and there is nothing more boring than heading for the sofa - again - when there are so many other more exciting things to do. I'm bored of being in the house so much while life continues elsewhere.

I'm bored of boring my friends with the endless symptoms: 'How you doing?' 'Oh, you know. I dropped a mug this morning. I tripped over the cat. I went to sleep. I had a bit of a wobble. How's you?' 'Well, after I partied all night, I had a fabulous day at work before whipping up a dinner party for eight. The usual.'

Then there's the boredom that comes with all the planning. MS is like a stroppy, badly-behaved toddler you have to lug around - for life. Before you go anywhere, you plan where the loos are, you work out if there's a café nearby to stop for a break, you pack a bag of stuff, you can't stay out too late.

When your world shrinks and spontaneity is something you have to think about seriously, there's not an awful lot of options left. Friends tire of always being bailed out on. I'm out of synch with them, going through an accelerated old age in my 30's.

The highlight of my day is getting a pen and marking an asterisk next to interesting programmes in the Radio Times. Years ago when I saw someone do this, I was scornful. How tragic, such an empty life. I mean, who does that? Um, well, me now.

So how can I combat this boredom? What can I do from the comfort and safety of my couch? Wordsearch puzzles? Solitaire? Spray-paint the cat purple?

19th March 2013

It's Not Working

When The Teenager was six, his class had to present a short talk about what their parents worked as. According to reports, he proudly announced to the class that 'My mummy studied for four years to become a psychopath and she has her own clinic where she sees people.'

A quick call from the school later, and I had reassured them that I was actually a homeopath. Some would say they're not dissimilar. Telling people you're a homeopath is akin to confessing you boil up frog skins and sulphur under a full moon, whilst chanting naked, trusted black cat by your side.

According to the media, we are a bunch of charlatans and confidence-tricksters who prey on vulnerable people. The recession and ill-health forced me to take a sabbatical from my clinic and I miss it. Homeopathy never felt like work, it was a passion and for me, it was always complementary, never an alternative to orthodox medicine.

I'm currently in the middle of looking for a new job. The builder can't employ me forever and much as I like stomping around in my Caterpillar boots, eating bacon sarnies, slurping tea and reading The Sun, it'll be time to move on soon.

Hours and hours of scrolling through countless job sites has left me shell-shocked and disheartened though. After putting in my location, the hours I want to work and my skill-set, I'm still only left with chambermaid, cleaner, carer and security guard jobs.

I know there's a recession on, but c'mon guys. So a little idea is slowly taking shape in my mind. I finish my degree in October, my head will be clear(ish) and I could possibly re-open my clinic. MS has altered my planned career-path, so why not combine the homeopathy with the knowledge gleaned from this degree in health and social care?

Hmm. If I had a brain, I'd be dangerous. I'd like to have a job where I could make a difference, however small. Not just working for the sake of it.

Anyway, it's just a thought for now. Who knows, my dream job may be just around the corner. Now excuse me while I light some incense sticks and pluck snails from my garden.

21st March 2013

Make Mine A Large One

With pleasure comes pain. The bacon butties and biscuits I have happily munched on since working for the builder have wreaked havoc on my figure, my muffin top morphing from a skinny raspberry into a full-blown, full-fat double chocolate chip with whipped cream on the side.

I had to face the awful reality that it was time for one of the most humiliating and sad events in any woman's life. Nope, I wasn't going to join a slimming club, I was going jeans shopping. Guaranteed to strike fear into the heart, I was going to be brave and thank my lucky stars that communal changing-rooms had been outlawed in the 1990's, along with shoulder pads, dodgy perms and ra-ra skirts.

And so I found myself wandering around shops where the sales assistants were young, hip and terrifyingly thin, showcasing the latest hot-off-the press fashion looks.

I furtively flicked through the rails, depressingly starting at the back where the larger sizes huddled in shame. A quick glance round and I shoved a couple of pairs over my arm, cleverly tucking the size labels inwards. Off to the changing room where a tiny sylph-like creature smirked as she slowly counted my items, handed me a plastic disc and waved me off to a cubicle towards the back.

Half an hour later, I was red-faced, exhausted and depressed. Whoever said skinny jeans suit everyone clearly lied. My MS balance (or lack of it) turned trying on five pairs of jeans into a farce. One leg in and I was pin-balling off the sides of the cubicle. Two legs in and I was jumping around like a hyperactive toddler on a pogo-stick.

When I could finally stand still, I was lucky enough to see my sorry figure from numerous angles thanks to eight different mirrors. I really do need to pick up that kettlebell for longer than three minutes at a time.

I found a pair I could live with, handed it over at the cash desk, not fooling the girl at all when I announced, 'Oh, I'm sure my friend will love these!' I left the store, turned a sharp right and headed for sanctuary. A coffee shop, where I ordered a large latte with an extra shot and the biggest muffin I could find.

23rd March 2013

Tripping All Over The Place

Did you know twice as many people die in trips and falls at home than in car crashes? No, me neither until I read the cheery news over breakfast yesterday. Now I have another thing to add to my list of worries that keep me awake in the wee small hours.

Foot drop is the bane of my life. I trip over flat surfaces, the cat, pavements, dust balls and just about anything else in my way. At Christmas I tripped up the stairs, then fell backwards, smashing into my bookcase and landing like a squashed spider on the floor, books raining down on me. The bruising was spectacular, but I did find a book I'd given up as lost.

There's no way of knowing when foot drop will strike. One day it leaves you in peace, the next it's shoving you around the high street with abandon. People give me a wide berth, as hey, I could be drunk. At 9.30 am.

Kerbs taunt me, potholes are a logistical nightmare when crossing the road and cobble-stones are pure evil. Sorry Shakespeare, but I am never, ever going to Stratford-upon-Avon ever again. A lovely little day trip turned into a day from hell when I got out the car and saw cobble-stones stretched out in every direction. I clung to my friend for dear life and quite possibly looked as if I was being taken out from a secure unit for the weekend as I muttered, 'evil, evil things, I hate you' under my breath every few minutes as he dragged me up the road.

Then there was the Gastro Pub Incident, when a friend took me out for dinner. A short stumble to the bathroom led to disaster as I cartwheeled across the floor in front of six bemused diners, ending up halfway under their table. To compound my misery, my friend hadn't even noticed as he was too busy scrolling through his phone. I limped back to our table, face burning, sniveling with pain and embarrassment.

Anyway, the good news is, the sixth most common way to die at home is by drowning in the bath. Thank you, MS heat intolerance for making baths a thing of the past. At least you're good for something.

25th March 2013

It's Only A Number. Isn't It?

Oh joy. I will be 39 plus 1 in less than half a year. I won't be celebrating, but rather I shall be holding a memorial service to my first 40 years, along with lashings of wine and copious amounts of cake.

To help me feel even more inadequate than usual, The Sunday Times Style magazine thoughtfully published a list of '40 Things To Do Before You're 40.' Here's some of the ones I haven't done and have no hope of doing before August:

- Get an accountant - ha ha thud. That's me laughing my head off?

- Bin all your tights and replace the lot with Falke - unfashionable me has no idea what/who Falke is. Hopeless.

- Have a kinky dream about a colleague - the builder? Seriously?

- Go to Glastonbury - nope.

- Host an afterparty that people still talk about years later - what the heck's an afterparty and why have I never been to one?

- Stop wearing lycra - never.

- Spend a year with an incredibly flat stomach - and give up Maltesers and toast? Crazy.

- Unwrap a diamond - not unless it's a Diamond White cider party pack.

- Grow your hair so long that it covers your nipples - one word - why?

But here's some I *have* done:

- Decide whether you want children - yup, I'm keeping the Teenager.

- Be able to order wine confidently - 'Cheapest bottle of your house white, and make it snappy, my good man.'

- Pull an all-nighter, drink Sambuca, dance on the tables, then go straight to work - too many times to mention.

- Live abroad long enough to get a taste for the local breakfast - those were the days. Sigh.

- Witness a birth - I was *definitely* there when The Teenager was born.

- Perfect your signature roast chicken - Waitrose, I love you.

Don't you just hate these lists? Here's my kind of list - recently-announced top 5 snacks in the UK (drum roll....) bacon butties came out top, no doubt helped along by my recent alarming consumption of them.

They were closely followed by cheese on toast, sausage rolls, Cornish pasties and Scotch eggs. Now that's a list you can get your teeth into.

29th March 2013

It's Beginning To Look A Lot Like Christmas

The shops are full of chocolate and cakes, magazines are stuffed with recipes, we've got two bank holidays and the kids are bouncing off the walls with excitement and e-numbers. Easter is rapidly turning into Christmas Mark II.

I'm not complaining. I love Easter. So much so that I put up my Easter branches (in lieu of a tree) weeks and weeks ago. I'm looking forward to lazing on my sofa watching 'Gone With The Wind' for the 27th time, pausing the telly only to hunt out more chocolate. (Handy hint for MSers - don't bother buying those teeny-weeny chocolate eggs wrapped in foil. If your hands are dodgy, like mine, the teeth-gnashing frustration really isn't worth the effort. Just buy several large ones instead).

Anyway, The Teenager is away for a week, so it's just me and the cat rattling around the house. The laundry basket is empty, the fridge is fully-stocked and I am going to use this time as a period of quiet reflection. I have decided to re-hash my New Year's resolutions, giving myself another chance to fail at unlocking my true potential.

My resolutions, in no particular order, are: eat less, exercise more, try new things and learn how to make a decent Hollandaise sauce. My emotional resolution is to stop being so hard on myself. I get frustrated and angry when MS fatigue drives me to the sofa yet again, when I bale out on friends or have to go to bed early.

I still raise my son, study, work and run a house, so maybe I should cut myself some slack. It's strange, but sometimes I forget I have MS. I just think, oh, that's the feet buzzing again or here comes the fatigue and whoops, nearly fell over there. It's become such a part of my life and it brings me up with a sharp shock when I think, 'oh yeah, I've got multiple sclerosis.'

So this Easter, with The Teenager away, I am going to indulge myself. I will be meeting up with friends (fingers crossed), reading trashy novels and magazines, trying out new recipes and chilling. I am going to be kind to myself, something I have really neglected to do recently. Happy Easter

6th April 2013

Single Parent, Multiple Sclerosis

Our little family has adjusted fairly well to life with multiple sclerosis, but now and again it throws up some major hurdles.

Even though my ex-husband and I are happily divorced and are bringing up The Teenager as well as we can despite the 140 mile distance between us, there are definitely times when it would be handy to have a partner around, or at least in the same city.

I'm booked in to hospital for my second round of Alemtuzumab treatment during the summer school holidays and it's coming round far too quickly. The Teenager will be at his dad's for a week as usual and with the way the dates have worked out this year, I will have just one full day to recover at home after three days in hospital before The Teenager is home again. I am panicking. Slightly.

Last year, the Alemtuzumab left me exhausted, weak and under the weather and I had several weeks sick leave from work but I also had three clear days on my own at home to start to recover.

I'm not so much worried about me, but about how The Teenager will feel seeing me lying on the sofa even more than usual. Is there anything more depressing than an ill parent? I tried to have a chat with him about it the other day and he's promised me that if I buy him enough pizza, he'll be fine, so here's my plan to get through the first week or so:

- Pizza

- Accept all offers of help

- When he's out with friends, have a sleep, so I'm fully(ish) awake when he's back

- Encourage/bribe The Teenager to have friends for sleepovers

- Stock the fridge with lots of good-quality ready-meals

- Ignore the dust

- Keep explaining that the treatment will ultimately make me much better in the long-term

- Pizza

My friend's daughter has offered to cat-and-house-sit again, so that's one less thing to worry about. I'll also organise a huge grocery delivery just before I go to hospital. I know what to expect this time round, so hopefully I'll be better prepared than last year.

I was feeling very chuffed with my list and plans, then I checked my diary again. Yup, I'll be turning 40 less than three weeks after the treatment. Now I really am panicking... (no small violins were harmed during writing this blog post)

12th April 2013

Basket Case

I'm not a fan of supermarket shopping and I should have been suspicious when The Teenager jumped at the chance to accompany me the other day.

I haven't given up online shopping, but my mum mentioned she had seen some artificial grass in a supermarket nearby and it was selling out fast.

It was one of those cut-price supermarkets - no frills, no helpful staff, prison-style strip lighting and pushy customers shoving their trolleys into any legs that had the audacity to get in their way of grabbing the last bottle of Lambrusco or tin of discounted baked beans.

'Muuuuuuuuuuuuuum, can I have a bag of doughnuts?'

'No.'

'Two doughnuts?'

'No.'

'One?' (sad face)

'Just let me find the blinking grass and we're out of here. What? Oh, alright then. ONE.'

I found the grass and tried to juggle four rolls of the stuff in my arms when The Teenager came back with a basket, one doughnut lying forlornly in the middle.

'Why do you need a basket for your donut?'

'Er. Um. Pepsi's cheap, only 25 pence a can and I never have pop and everyone else in school has pop in the house and it's not fair that everyone else in school gets to have pop and I don't and I really think it's so cheap that it would be really nice if for once I could have some pop in the house so I'm just like all my friends and won't feel so different from everyone else. See?'

'Oh really?'

'Yeah. Pleeeeeeaaaaaasssssse? Just say 'stop' at the number of cans I can have? Tennineeightsevensixfivefourthree...'

'THREE. You can have three. One a day for the next three days as a treat. Then it's checkout.'

We queue up, offload the grass, Pepsi and solitary doughnut.

'Muuuuuuuum'.

'No.'

'You don't even know what I was going to say.'

'Yes. I. Do.'

'Awwwwww. Can I just get one tiny packet of chewing gum? Everyone else in school gets to have chewing gum and....'

'STOP. Don't go any further. I know exactly what you're going to say. I'm your mum. I'm a mind-reader.'

'Meanie.'

'Right, put the doughnut and the Pepsi back then.'

And so on and so on. And that is yet another good reason for never, ever going supermarket shopping.

14th April 2013

'D' Is For Cog Fog

I am a dunce. No two ways about it, MS has seriously fogged up my brain.

I first noticed it before I was diagnosed - simple recipes became infuriating Mensa-like tests, I got lost driving to the shops and reading a book was an exercise in tedious endurance.

I'm in my final year of my part-time degree and the last five years have been pretty good. I'm an unabashed girly swot and enjoy cracking open a new packet of Sharpies, drawing intricate mind maps, carefully crafting my essays, ferreting out incisive references.

Then my brain went on holiday with a one-way ticket. After an agonising couple of weeks last month, I finally submitted my first essay of my final year. The mind maps never moved beyond a bunch of circles with nothing in them and my Sharpies lay dormant.

I got my result yesterday. It was 65%. Sigh. Such a sad, sad little number. I normally get higher marks, so this was upsetting but not totally unexpected. I often struggle to add up simple numbers or find the right word, so writing a 2,500 essay is akin to scaling Mount Everest in flip-flops.

In the middle of recounting a funny anecdote to friends over coffee, my mind can go completely blank, the punchline withering and dying as my friends look at me with pity.

I read recently that memory loss is the most commonly reported cognitive difficulty in MS. Last year, when I was revising for my exam, I had written up a set of comprehensive study notes. They were a thing of beauty. I read them over and over and over again, but nothing, not one tiny thing, would stick inside my brain. I barely scraped through the three hour exam but luckily my fabulous MS nurse wrote a letter to the university explaining that I was not stupid, it was the MS.

My next essay is due at the end of May and I'm hoping for some divine inspiration. In the meantime, I'm furiously highlighting points in my books, jotting down what I hope will be valid arguments and crossing my fingers for luck. And no, the Sharpies haven't been used yet, but they're on my desk, raring to go. How do I draw a mind map again?

20th April 2013

Getting On My Nerves

It's been a stressful week and stress plus MS equals a spike in symptoms. I have tried everything to stay serene and in control - deep breathing, chocolate, mindfulness, two episodes of Mad Men.

The deep breathing made me feel a bit silly, the chocolate nudged the scales up, the 'Power of Now' was the 'Power of Not-Right-Now' and as for Mad Men, well, two episodes are never enough.

For me, it's mostly an increase in nerve pain. Ever tried describing nerve pain to the uninitiated? Burning, tingling, numbness, crawling, aching doesn't even begin to cover it. Tingling sounds delightful, numbness sounds painless, crawling sounds weird and we all ache, don't we? Just like we all get tired.

It's been driving me round the twist all week and as always with MS, it doesn't come alone. It's the great MS special offer - have one symptom, get three free'. So, as well as the nerve pain, there's the fatigue, the wonkier walking, the hands that'd be better suited to a Greek taverna. Smashed plates? Yup, as well as my last proper grown-up wine glass and yet another chip in yet another bowl.

I lay awake most of last night listening to the cat miaow loudly. For a tiny cat, she's got a huge set of lungs. The

Teenager got up and shut his door and I was left to ponder the cobwebs on the ceiling and listen to a group of drunk woman sing 'Simply the Best' outside my window at 1.30 am.

The pain was excruciating and made even more unbearable as my legs started to jerk and twitch. I wasn't sure if it was like being possessed by a malevolent spirit (The Exorcist sprang to mind in the wee small hours) or being stretched on a rack. Only problem was, I couldn't get up and go downstairs as the cat would think it was perfectly normal to sit in the kitchen listening to the shipping forecast before sunrise.

I was trapped and the women outside moved on to a Tom Jones medley, a tortuous backdrop to insane pain. Action plan for the weekend - rescue 'The Power of Now' book from the corner I flung it in to, lie on the sofa with a huge bag of crisps and a relaxing face-pack on and chant, 'this too shall pass' over and over and over again.

30th April 2013

A Back-Handed Compliment

'But you look so well.' A loaded sentence most of us with MS hear at some point.

I hear it a lot, along with 'but I heard you were ill'. The complex nature of my, so far, mostly hidden illness. What they don't see is the work that goes on behind the scenes. Yes, I look fine for that hour or so. No, they don't see me taking ages to get ready or lying on the sofa afterwards. Or the long evenings spent alone at home, too tired to go out with friends.

I'm proud that I still want to look my best, but not fitting the physical perception of the 'sick role' can distort the view people have of me. I'm used to it, or so I thought until Saturday.

I was at an MS meeting. At the end of it, we gathered around in groups for a coffee. I was talking to a friend when suddenly a woman I had never seen before pushed in and without any greeting, asked if I had MS. 'Um, yes?' She looked me up and down before saying, 'but you look so well.'

It was the 'but' that threw me. She didn't say, 'great to see you looking so well' or ask how long I had been diagnosed. I felt immediately guilty, as if I had to justify myself. I had always thought that I was 'safe' with other people with MS - no need to explain nerve pain, fatigue or the general fed-upness that goes with MS.

I told her that I had been having relapse after relapse and had been offered Campath (Alemtuzumab) treatment and touch wood, no relapses since last May. 'Relapses? Hah. I never had any' she said. 'Oh. Is that good?' 'No! I've just gone downhill. I have primary progressive MS. We don't have any miracle cures. Nothing can be done for us, all the research, all the meds go on the ones with relapsing remitting MS.'

Awkward. What do you say to that? I made my excuses and wandered away. I wasn't in the mood to be challenged. I went home deflated and upset. I did see it from her viewpoint, but it was the abruptness of the exchange that threw me.

I don't want to justify myself to other people with MS. I have to do it enough to everyone else. I went home, dragged my duvet onto the sofa and fell asleep. 4pm and the day was over.

3rd May 2013

The Return of The Angry Red Tomato-Face

Men in loud-patterned shorts and sandals are everywhere, I have a stack of special offer leaflets from supermarkets urging me to stock up on barbecue essentials and the weather forecasters can barely contain their excitement. We are having a spell of warm, sunny weather and I am not best pleased.

In fact, I'm downright grumpy. Two years ago I enjoyed the warm weather as much as anyone, but one day that all changed as my face morphed into an angry red blur, my limbs went weak and I felt faint with fatigue. Since then Uhthoff's phenomenon, otherwise known as heat intolerance, has made my life a misery.

A tiny spot of sun will add a youthful, flushed glow to my face. Any more than that and I begin to scare small children. I often wish I was born 100 years ago so I could carry a parasol when outdoors and recline on a chaise-lounge, delicately fluttering a fan and sipping peppermint tea when the heat gets too much. And a bonnet would be ideal for bad hair days.

It's not just weather that does this - hot radiators in the winter, 'atmospheric' log fires in gastropubs and over-heated shops all take their toll. Opening the oven door is a tricky operation. Do it too quickly and I've got to lie down for five minutes, food sadly forgotten. I fondly remember giving myself home-made facials by adding lavender to a

bowl of boiling water and steaming my face over it.
Nowadays that would probably be the best way to make
me give up my PIN numbers and passwords.

I am now a semi-vampire, hiding in the house as much
as I can and my super-size fan is my new best friend. I
have become an expert at judging where any breeze is
coming from. I rearrange chairs in cafés when a blast of
sun comes through the window.

So this bank holiday weekend, I will mostly be at home.
I will not be going to a barbecue - it's insanity to cook in
the heat. I will not be going to the beach. I will not be
sitting outside a pub. I will instead smile through gritted
teeth when yet another person says, 'oooh, lovely weather
we're having!' Isn't it just.

7th May 2013

Would (Not) Like To Meet

To cheer myself up at the weekends, I read the dating columns in the newspapers, especially the upmarket ones. I also chortle over the birth announcements in The Times: Oscar-Theodore Chummingly-Wallop, a brother for Broccoli-Cressida and Seraphina-Arabella has a different ring to it than Kev, a brother for Chelsee and Kaycee.

My least favourite dating advert is the one that starts, 'my secretary said, don't mention the distant travel, restaurants and fine hotels, just say you are kind and successful and seeking a younger lady up to the age of 40.' What decade is this guy living in? The one where women knew their place and how to mix a mean Martini with a twist, whilst whipping up a three-course dinner when hubby's boss unexpectedly invites himself to dinner?

I love the show-offs - the 'Cambridge University educated gentleman, 70's' (get over yourself dear, you graduated half a century ago), 'London or Paris, loves jazz' (bless him, he went on a Eurostar day trip years ago) and 'ohac, 80' (honestly, I would *hope* he'd have his own home and car at that age).

Then there are the downright odd. 'Attractive, professional businessman, lives near cliffs'. I'd be worried. 'Divorced, 63, own teeth and hair, with no beard or tattoos or earrings but a gsoh'. There are no words.

There're also the 'humorous' ones - 'Detached and desirable and much sought after luxury property. All mod cons, in full working order, circa 1950's. Early viewing essential!' Gosh, I bet he's a right barrel of laughs.

I have learned that most of the men go to the theatre and enjoy good food. Does anyone enjoy bad food? The majority of them are looking for someone slim and younger than they are. They like golf and classic cars and seem to be solvent, apart from the man who boldly states that 'I believe the best things in life are free'. Ladies, steer clear.

To be fair, I have also 'written' my own advert - 'Single, divorced parent to a sulky Teenager and bonkers cat, late 30's. Tall, has MS'. I bet I'd be inundated...

9th May 2013

But Is It Art?

It was a lovely plan - a day spent at the art gallery. I imagined myself wandering around (artistically), lost in thought, occasionally throwing out deep and insightful comments to my companion in reverential, hushed tones. He would be impressed by the breadth of my knowledge, adding musings of his own. Afterwards, we would sit in the café and contemplate the wondrous art we had seen over double-shot espressos and hand-crafted scones.

I guess we just weren't in the mood. We scooted through the galleries, stopping short at odd, randomly-placed sculptures before moving on to the modern art section. We whizzed past each picture: 'Nah.' 'What's that supposed to be?' 'The Teenager could do better than that.' 'Hey, check this out, it's supposed to represent the dichotomy of suffering in an existential landscape' (a canvas with two blobs on it).

'Wow, this guy was pretty radical, he painted the frame too.' 'Lunch?' 'Yeah, let's go.'

We ended up by the coast and looked out over the sea whilst waiting for the restaurant to open. My friend had a mischievous grin as he started bouncing in the seat of his wheelchair. 'Seagull! Want seagull!' 'Shut up, people are looking.' 'Ice cream, ice cream, ice cream, ice cream.' 'Shhhhhhh. People are staring.' 'That's the whole point. They probably think there's something wrong with me

anyway, sitting in a wheelchair. Wanna go on the boat.
Boat, boat, boat. '

Thankfully, lunch passed without incident and we
discussed everything and nothing about living with MS and
whether it was acceptable to poke fun at ourselves and our
disabilities. We decided to round off the afternoon with a
coffee. Queuing up, that mischievous glint returned to his
eye. In a loud voice he announced 'Aww, you're the best
carer I've ever had.'

10th May 2013

Stumbling In Crutches

I am feeling rather sorry for myself. As I write, there is a pair of crutches next to me and I am floating among pink, fluffy clouds thanks to the strong painkillers.

Yesterday I fell quite badly, and to be fair, it wasn't due to the MS, it was me not looking where I was going. Unfortunately though, my MS treatment has left me with a tendency to have out-of-proportion bruising, so my leg is now a fabulous riot of colours and has swollen so much I can't get my jeans on.

To top it off, I think the shock of it has increased my nerve pain temporarily so I'm buzzing and tingling all over. The bruising must be impressive as The Teenager keeps wanting a look at it, saying 'ewwwwwww' before taking another look. All in all, not the best of days.

Thank goodness for family and friends. My partner-in-crime at the museum trip came up trumps and after making numerous phone calls, tracked down a pair of crutches I can borrow. My mum is carting away loads of laundry for me and drops round food supplies, flowers and news of the outside world.

So, yet again, I am whiling away the hours at home, not studying, not writing up my essay notes and chomping obscene amounts of Maltesers and Bacon Bites. Ho hum.

I have worked out how to switch on the fire with a crutch without getting off the sofa, I count down the hours to my next lot of painkillers and The Teenager has had two takeaways in a row. I'd like to say I have learnt something from this experience, that I will never, ever take my health for granted, but hey, didn't I just go through all this recently with the whole MS saga?

I don't need any more time out to re-evaluate the direction of my life. Been there, done that, drowned my sorrows. So I'm off to have another pity party and pop more painkillers. My mum is at the supermarket buying me a tub of prunes. Life goes on.

12th May 2013

How To Lose Friends And Alienate People

Having something as serious as MS enter your life changes it forever. Family, work, future plans, and of course, health. Sadly, it also lets you find out who your true friends are. Right from the start, cherished friends deserted my sinking ship just when I needed them most. Some left abruptly without a backwards glance, others backed away slowly, step by step.

Why? I guess there are many reasons. Were they worried they'd be roped into looking after me? Would I rely on them more than usual? Were we now too different, too alienated from each other to have much in common anymore?

Conversely, other friends rose to the challenge - they stuck by me through everything. They listened to me rant and rave, they wiped my tears, poured my wine and probably ended up knowing more about MS than they could ever have imagined.

Two years on, I thought nothing else could surprise me. I have a fantastic circle of friends and I hope I'm a good friend to them too, and as the MS crisis has receded, our relationship has re-balanced itself. A couple of weeks ago, my world was rocked once more.

An old friend got back in touch. We met years ago in work and although we only kept in touch sporadically, we always picked up where we left off. We chatted by text and I suggested he look at my blog to catch up with everything that had happened since we last spoke. And that was the last I heard from him.

I feel hurt. Actually, I feel extremely hurt. And angry. The ripples and repercussions from MS are still going on, two years down the line. Now I'm semi-housebound once more after falling last week, I have too much time on my hands to reflect on this. And do you know what? It's all good.

Those 'friends' who've left have made way for even better friends. They took their hang-ups and made space for new friends to fill the void. If any of my friends ever face a situation like I have and I'm not sure how to handle it, the least I can say is, 'I don't know what to do or say, but I am here for you, you know that.' And that is the mark of a real friend.

14th May 2013

Livin' La Vida Sofa

Since my spectacular fall last week, I have been hobbling around at home going stir crazy. I made a break for freedom on Sunday when a friend enticed me outside with the offer of brunch and some retail therapy. He quickly walked ahead of me as I yelled, 'Hello trees! Hello shops! I'm out!' and grinned manically at everyone I passed in the street.

Two hours later he dropped me back home, full of coffee but exhausted. My leg was throbbing and as I peeled my jeans off the bruise spread even further. Oops. I have a sinking feeling the injury will take a lot longer to heal than I first thought. I'm not going anywhere this week, so I skulk around the house and spend far too much time on my sofa.

When The Teenager comes home from school, I bribe him with cake in the vain hope he will sit down long enough to tell me what it's like in the outside world but all he wants to do is have another look at my bruise before heading upstairs to tweet and get up to the next level of Candy Crush.

I have set up a Command Centre from my sofa - everything I need is within reach. Remote control, magazines, mobile phone, Bacon Bites. I have watched every programme on my Sky Planner and now have to resort to watching Catherine Cookson adaptations and angry people shouting at each other on Jeremy Kyle. Friends and family have been brilliant. My mum comes round every day with gossip and my latest batch of laundry. A friend dropped off a huge Victoria sponge on Saturday.

Even the cat is behaving, although we argue over duvet rights on the sofa. My days are punctuated by painkillers and chocolate (it's medicinal). I really should get cracking on my next essay. I need to put an online shopping order in. My bank statements are staring at me from my desk. The dust balls are having a party and my garden is sadly neglected.

Life is on hold. I remain optimistic though. MS has taught me to expect the unexpected. Soon enough, things will return to normal. In the meantime, a friend is coming over soon with the new issue of Grazia and I'm going to chuck the cat off my duvet. Again.

16th May 2013

Do You Suffer From MS? I Don't.

Guaranteed to set my teeth on edge, the term 'MS sufferer' is up there with 'But you look so well' and 'Oh, I get tired too.' It makes for good copy - by starting an article with, 'MS sufferer Mrs Jones....blah blah blah', the reader is immediately directed to feel a certain way - pity, thank god it's not me, poor thing.

Well, here's the real news - I don't want to be pitied. I don't want anyone to look at me with big, sad eyes or vicariously imagine how awful my life is. The media have a lot to answer for.

Most of us who live with MS fly under the radar. We get on with life, we hold down jobs, we raise families, we cope. We don't want to be lumped together in a mass of misery. It's similar to the pressure people with cancer can feel under to 'fight back' against their illness and if they 'fail', well, they fought a brave battle, didn't they?

Perhaps because MS is at present incurable, we are not urged to fight back, just suffer instead, hopefully in silence. I am many things. A daughter, a mother, a colleague, a student, a friend. I also happen to have MS, I just don't feel the need to qualify the term. I'm not saying life with MS is easy. It's anything but. Yet by labeling me a sufferer, I am instantly at a disadvantage, pushed into the role of a hapless victim, MS being the only defining feature of an otherwise fulfilling life.

So how should we be known? Well, it depends on the context. If someone is talking about me as a mother, then I'm a mother, not a 'mother suffering from MS'. If it's about my job, then I'd like to be known as an excellent worker, not 'working despite suffering from MS.' And if the conversation is simply about MS, then just call me a 'person with MS'. Or if you want to be really kind, 'that fabulous person with MS'....

22nd May 2013

Haematoma Blues (And Purples, And Reds...)

My magnificent bruising has been reclassified as a haematoma, which probably explains why I'm still hobbling around two weeks since my accident. I was lucky enough to see one of our fabulous MS nurses at a Work and MS conference on Saturday and during a coffee break, I rolled my jeans down in the loos to show her the injury. She carefully examined it and suggested I take myself off to Accident and Emergency to have it scanned in case there was an underlying fracture.

To cut a long story short, my mum took me that evening and the good news is, it's just a haematoma, not a fracture. The bad news is, the only thing I can do is wait for the swelling to go down. It's not going anywhere fast and neither am I.

The pace of my life wasn't particularly speedy before (take a bow, MS fatigue and foot drop) but has now slowed to a virtual stop. I've been told to keep my leg elevated as much as possible, so needing no excuse to lie down and fill my brain with trashy t.v. when I should be slaving over an essay, my sofa is now almost permanently in use, much to the chagrin of the cat.

The Teenager marvels at my easy life and prods the lump on my leg in wonder. He's very much enjoying visiting friends for tea after school and has perfected his tragic face when talking to their parents, 'oh, my mum's dreadfully ill, she's got this massive thing on her leg, the size of a rugby ball, honestly, she can barely speak, it's that bad' before gratefully accepting yet another chocolate roll or can of Coke.

I'm sure I'll be back on my feet soon enough and will no doubt look back wistfully on my weeks at home when I go back to work. But I do miss the banter and bacon rolls and even my nickname, 'Half-Shift'...

24th May 2013

Transformation. Complete?

Tomorrow it will be exactly a year since I was unceremoniously ushered out of the MS Limboland waiting room and into a whole new world of clinically definite multiple sclerosis.

MS has had an impact upon every area of my life. Everything has been transformed and I'm not the same person I was last May, but for my MS anniversary, I am going to concentrate on the positive changes.

I've done my grieving, I've cried myself hoarse. I could either live out a sad, bitter life, railing against the injustice of it all or seize this opportunity to change my life for the better.

I'm full of gratitude for the support network I have - the family and friends who stuck by me through the dark times. The ones who made a swift exit? Probably for the best, eh? I'm indebted to all the healthcare staff who pulled me through and who continue to support me and I've made a whole new circle of brilliant friends.

Being bullied at work and subsequently sacked simply for having MS showed me that when I'm pushed into a corner, I can still come out fighting. Ironically, as my colleagues were trying to crush my spirit, the whole experience made me stronger, braver and has restored my self-esteem.

Probably the biggest transformation though, is within my own character. I'm no longer willing to live a life according to what is 'normal' or what is expected of me. I am choosing my own path. For far too long I have gone through life reacting to the whims and actions of other people, forgetting in all the chaos that in fact, I had a choice all along.

It took something far bigger than those people to turn my world upside down and to put into perspective just how fleeting and how beautiful life is. MS is here to stay, for now, and as long as it does, we have to learn to get along. It's part of me, so I can't hate it. I have to keep learning to adapt, take the good days with the bad. Is the transformation complete? You betcha. Phase One at least.

28th May 2013

MS - A Life Of Opposites

MS is a bizarre illness - there are hundreds of combinations of symptoms and no one person's MS is the same as another's. It's like an MS pick-n-mix, except MS does the choosing.

What's most frustrating though is the sheer contradiction in symptoms. One day I'll have all the windows open, the fan going at full blast, an arctic wind whipping round my feet. The next, I'm chilled to the bone, wrapped in my duvet clutching my hot water bottle.

Or there's the foot-drop - the days when my feet decide to do an Irish jig and every pavement becomes a minefield, in sharp contrast to other days when my legs are rigid and I walk like a wound-up robot. On top of that is my old nemesis, MS fatigue, the bane of my life. Striking at any time, it drives me to my sofa, everything else on hold until normal service resumes. So why do I also have periods of extreme insomnia? Nights when I sit downstairs listening to the World Service.

It's not just the physical symptoms - my emotions swing from one extreme to the other too. On Sunday I was feeling on top of the world but on Monday I had one of my gloomy days. Nothing had happened to explain it. Perhaps it is the daily pressure of trying to maintain a normal life while coping with the whole MS thing, who knows?

I'm off to the Hay-on-Wye book festival with friends today, a trip I've been looking forward to for months. Apart from the haematoma on my leg which is still as painful as ever, I'm praying that the fatigue also takes a day trip, in the opposite direction.

I'm hoping it won't be a day when I just want to go back to bed, pull my duvet over me and shut out the world. MS can be a very unsociable illness and not knowing from one day to the next just what it'll throw at you makes life even more difficult to plan, but for today, I am going out whether MS likes it or not. So if you're in Hay-on-Wye today and see a chubby-faced woman fast asleep on a deckchair, that'll be me.

30th May 2013

Mixing With The Literati

With Bill Clinton once describing it as the 'Woodstock of the mind', I was over-excited to visit the Hay-on-Wye Book Festival on Tuesday.

Months ago, a friend and I had booked tickets for our kids to see one of their favourite authors and so we headed up through the damp Welsh countryside to the London literary outpost for a day of intellectual thought, musings and trying to grab the last seat in the café as we sheltered from the thundering rain.

The Teenager was suitably impressed that his talk would be held in the Google-sponsored tent (result) and at home later told me in reverential, hushed tones that the author had been 'mint' and had inspired him to read more (another result).

Anyway, we wandered around and settled down in the tented area for a picnic lunch, eschewing the over-priced venison burgers and alfalfa salad. I was dismayed to note that almost everyone, and I really do mean everyone, was in Hunter wellies and green wax jackets. My own boots were letting in water and squelched every time I walked. Children with long, wild hair were happily munching on cucumber batons and holding onto their crowns, made in the kids craft tent.

Our kids, on the other hand, made a nuisance of themselves by pilfering the free cheese samples, going back again and again, claiming they needed yet another freebie for various fictional elderly relatives. With two of our kids safely offloaded into the Google tent, we had a coffee, having sneaked into the 'Friends' tent.

Apparently if you pay £25, you get priority booking and have a special 'Friends' queue at each event, a kind of highbrow 'Fast-Track' ticket like those you can buy at amusement parks. 'Friends' proudly displayed their special ID badges and elbowed past us at high speed.

It's suitably apt that Hay is twinned with Timbuktu. It really was an out of the world, strange experience. Apparently the late singer-songwriter Ian Dury rewrote the lyrics to 'Hit Me With Your Rhythm Stick' at Hay in one of his last concerts - the famous line reading, 'From the gardens of Babylon, all the way to lovely Hay.'

We ended our great day with chips from the chippy made famous by the DJ Chris Evans, who marvelled at the fact they use a spray gun to slather the chips in vinegar. Who says we ain't highbrow?

31st May 2013

What Not To Say To Someone With MS

When I was going through the whole MS diagnostic process, people said the strangest (and hurtful) things to me. It was hard enough coming to terms with MS, far less finding smart replies to insensitive comments.

Everyone has an opinion and they can't wait to give it to you. Even after diagnosis, the comments still keep coming, perhaps because MS is, for now, a mostly invisible illness for me and trying to convey the symptoms to other people is as difficult as counting brain lesions without an MRI.

So here's my handy print-out-and-keep list of what not to say to someone with MS. Give it to all your newly-diagnosed friends to prepare them for the onslaught and before long, they'll have ticked every one, several times over:

- You need to stay positive.

- You'll be fine, they can do wonders these days.

- My auntie/friend/great-uncle Billy had that, and they're great now.

- When are you giving up work?

- I've heard Diet Coke and chewing gum can give you MS.

- You get to sleep a lot? Wow, great symptom, wish I had that.

- Hey, it could be worse.

- But you look so good!

- If you get a blue badge, can I borrow it?

- Have you tried (insert any number of miracle cures here...)?

- You're so brave.

- You're cancelling our evening out...AGAIN??

- At least you don't actually look disabled.

- You're not using that old MS excuse again, are you?

So what should they say? Best piece of advice is not to presume things, just ask me questions. Ask what it means to me and my life. Everyone's MS is different. And if you don't know what to say, say nothing. Just give me a hug and crack open the chocolate.

2nd June 2013

Pause. Press Play

After more than three weeks off work with a lumpy haematoma on my leg, I am finally off my sofa and raring to go.

When I tell people I work for my builder friend, they raise an eyebrow, look me up and down and say, 'Oh, really?' They might have visions of me driving a large white van, chucking plasterboard around and fitting worktops in my spare time.

Years ago when I helped my friend set up his company, this was probably true. He taught me how to use a drill and I became an excellent tiler. Those days are long gone, although I can still tile if I sit on a bench and the boss applies the adhesive for me first. It's a bit like mosaic craft work. Until the tiles fall off.

My boss is the Patron Saint of Hopeless Causes and reluctantly agreed to let me work with him after I was sacked from my job. I begged, cajoled and consented to listening to commercial radio all day long. Obviously MS has put paid to most of the things I used to do, so we have 'adapted and overcome'. Well, I have. The boss may well disagree.

So now, my duties consist of - making tea and coffee, putting the radio on, tidying up the boss's toolbox, sweeping things in to little piles everywhere (which I then trip over), gossiping, yelling out a countdown to lunchtime, making more tea and coffee and spending hours nattering to the owners of whichever house we are working on (or 'skiving', as the boss calls it)

If there's a job where my presence is more of a hindrance, I work from home, writing up quotes, sourcing materials and helping him with his website, so I'm not completely useless. When I asked the boss if he had missed me when I was off, he looked bemused and paused mid-way through drilling. 'Missed what?' I flounced (limped and stumbled) off, but he has a point, I suppose.

He rattled off the facts - 'you keep dropping the nails, you trip over everything, I find you dozing off in quiet corners, you can't lift anything heavier than a hammer, and you talk non-stop. What's to miss?'

4th June 2013

Driving Miss Crazy

The day I was diagnosed with MS I was instructed to inform the Driver and Vehicle Licensing Agency (DVLA) toot suite, on pain of flogging or death. Well, no, not really, but it was a pretty stern diktat.

I duly found my way through their labyrinth website, downloaded the forms and sent them off. A year passed and I was confident they had forgotten all about me and had guessed I was still a safe driver. I had even taken an ice and snow driving course when I lived in Norway, a terrifying day where I drove down a vertical hill covered in oil to simulate the experience.

The other week though I received a letter with the words, 'the Medical Advisor has recommended that your current licence is withdrawn...and a new licence will be issued to you, which will be only be valid for 3 years.' Bearing in mind my previous licence was valid until well into the 2040's, I was a bit upset.

For unscientific research purposes, I asked the Twittersphere if this was a standard procedure. Apparently it is. Which strikes me as rather odd and arbitrary. If only the powers that be who will be overseeing the change from Disability Living Allowance (DLA) to the Personal Independence Payment (PIP) could also accept that MS is a degenerative, progressive illness with no cure. Why make us re-prove that we have MS and it doesn't get better? I doubt that anyone with MS who has a 3 year license will suddenly be deemed 'cured' and re-issued with a longer licence.

To rub salt into the wound, I am also now banned from driving 3.5 - 7.5 tonne vehicles and minibuses (not for hire or reward), for medical reasons. Not that I have any intention of doing so, but it would have been nice to have had the choice.

So now my licence lasts until 2016 at which point they will review my case. I'm off out now for a little tootle in the car. The Thermos is ready, the tartan blanket is packed and I have a tin of pear drops in the glove compartment. Just to be on the safe side.

7th June 2013

Party Pooper

I have two family gatherings in the next couple of days. I love my family to pieces and adore spending time with them. That's not the problem. It's the uninvited guest who always tags along with me that's giving me palpitations. MS hisses in my ear, 'you can't go, you'll be too tired, too hot, too tingly, too boring - why don't you just go back to your sofa, have a nice lie down.'

I am an awkward guest now, like the Mad Aunt everyone knows they have to invite but aren't quite sure what to do with. Chairs and parasols are rearranged in the garden thanks to heat intolerance, guests look away politely as I spill my drink thanks to dodgy hands and my jokes fall flat as I suddenly can't remember all-important punchlines thanks to cog fog.

Don't get me wrong, my family are wonderful, it's just that MS has driven an invisible wedge between us. Sitting in a dark, shady corner watching everyone else bask in the sun is a metaphor for life with MS.

So, I have some pre-prepared answers ready to lessen the awkwardness and make me appear slightly less tragic: 'You keep yawning, are we keeping you up?' - 'Hell no, was out last night dancing on the tables, fabulous time, wasn't back 'til 2 am' 'Hey, come out into the sun!!' - 'S'ok, Vogue said pale is the new tan' 'Whoops, careful' -

'No worries, it takes skill you know, to trip over a flat surface and I'm the champion'

Good plan, no? My family all know I have MS but I don't really want to belabour the point, and as most of us with MS know, trying to describe the symptoms is not for party-talk, it's a full-blown maudlin evening over wine, Pringles, low-burning candles and Edith Piaf in the background.

And anyway, I feel awkward enough without wanting everyone else to feel the same way too. So I will try my hardest. I will take part in pass-the-new-baby-around, but perhaps pass him on a little quicker than the others. I will grip my wine glass with two hands, as if I am drinking from a chalice. I will pinch some ice cubes and surreptitiously pop them down my top. Above all, I will attempt to leave my uninvited guest at the door, just for a while.

10th June 2013

The Venerable Order of the Uhthoff Vampires

Uhthoff's Phenomenon (try saying that without sounding like a muppet singing 'Mahna Mahna') is a serious problem for lots of us with MS, where heat can worsen our neurological symptoms. I am therefore establishing 'The Venerable Order of the Uhthoff Vampires' and anyone who's familiar with the following scenarios is cordially invited to claim free membership:

- When that big shiny yellow thing in the sky appears, you shake a fist at it before slinking back into the shadows.

- You have bought (and discarded) numerous hand-held fans but feel a bit daft using one in public.

- When a friend suggests a bit of sun-bathing at the beach, you're sorely tempted to whack them over the head with their flip-flops.

- The very thought of having a sauna is torture and you'd rather pull out your eyelashes one by one.

- You quite fancy a nice holiday in Iceland or the Antarctic.

- You're idea of bliss is to open your freezer and stick your head inside.

For the uninitiated, heat intolerance is like pouring hot oil over already-damaged brain circuits. MS means your nerves don't fire messages properly, but with a bit of luck, they'll eventually get through. Add a dose of heat on top of this and you get serious meltdown.

My body collapses in on itself, my struggling brain shuts up shop and I go a peculiar shade of pillar-box red. In the summer, my days are topsy-turvey. I get up around 5 am and stumble around doing as much as possible before the dreaded sun starts shining.

Then I lurk at home, fan at full blast until early evening when I suddenly come alive again. Or not, if MS fatigue decides to join forces with Evil Uhthoff and create a lethal combination.

I spend hours peering through my windows watching carefree sun-worshippers stroll past, taunting me with their tans, their bright summer clothes and languid chatter. When people visit my tiny haven of a backyard, they admire the plants and hand-made pottery toadstools then remark, 'shame you don't get much sunlight here though.' Um, exactly?'

So join me in the shadows. Don't lurk alone. Vampires are bang on-trend. Just look at Edward Cullen and his Twilight buddies (I do, a lot, much to The Teenager's eternal embarrassment).

14th June 2013

Job Hunting Just Got Uglier

Oh marvellous. As if job hunting with a disability in a recession isn't hard enough, beautifulpeople.com launched their own recruitment service last month, an offshoot of their dating agency for people who are beautiful and (boy, do they) know it. Really.

40,000 members have already signed up and last week 60 employers posted vacancies in a single 48-hour period. What hope is there for the rest of us? I may as well rip up my CV, stick a paper bag over my head and find a job peeling sacks of potatoes in my local chip shop.

There is an interesting interview with the Beautiful Fran, a member who claims 'a slick of tinted moisturiser and some light eye make-up are all the products I need to ensure I look beautiful.' Well, I've had a look at her photo and I've seen less make-up on a drag queen, but who am I to judge?

Fran boldly states that 'looks now play a part in every profession.' A sweeping, untrue comment, but then this is the same woman who also says that 'it's a fact that women judge each other on their appearance.' Oh really? You might do that, love, but in the real world, it's a fact that most of us quite simply don't.

What really annoys me though is when she says, '...women were obviously jealous of me (in an office) and they would say nasty things behind my back - and even sometimes to my face.' In my humble opinion, I would say this happened more because of her arrogant attitude and the way she interacts with other women rather than her perceived beauty.

If she thinks *that's* discrimination, what on earth is she doing joining a website that proudly and blatantly discriminates? Workplace bullying is a serious problem and having been through it myself for a year, I find it insulting that she even mentions this.

I don't think I've been hit too badly with the ugly stick, but when I go for job interviews I hope I can convey a passion and knowledge for the role rather than worrying if I've got hair on my lip gloss. Looks fade but insight and wisdom only grow over the years. Fran's got an answer to this though. She's considering Botox...

22ⁿᵈ June 2013

Keep It. Store It. Chuck It

As I approach an, ahem, milestone birthday (stop sniggering at the back) I took a long hard look around my house and finally decided to put my student years behind me.

I faced up to the fact that my attempt to channel a New York loft vibe was just never going to work in a tiny, 160 year old cottage in Wales. Every corner was stuffed with random artwork, quirky finds, mismatched crockery, a growing Teenager and a cat. Something had to give.

So I put the cat up for adoption. No, not really, but I wanted a clear-out, a fresh start, preferably without resorting to hiring a chanting shaman to wander round the house burning bundles of sage.

Yesterday, my ruthless mission was completed. Every single item in the house has been thoroughly assessed - keep, store or chuck. That sewing machine I bought with the whimsical notion of spending delightful evenings running up curtains, Cath Kidston duvet covers and cute little jam pot covers? Donated to a friend. The crafting glue gun stays however, for the sheer comedy factor. Hours of fun guaranteed.

My books were culled, boxed up and stored in the attic. I took down half my pictures and paintings, ornaments were decimated and I got rid of the sofa in my bedroom. I rifled through my wardrobe, trying on everything and parting company with all the clothes I was keeping just in case I magically lost three stone. If that miracle ever did occur, believe me, I would write begging letters to Gok Wan, pleading with him to help me find my new fashion direction.

MS has been a great opportunity to audit my entire life from top to bottom, but it's not always been as much fun as deciding whether a 'novelty' toothbrush holder can stay or go. My career path has altered drastically, cherished friends have disappeared overnight and I'm still finding my way in this brave new world.

From the depths of despair though, my life is being rebuilt and I won't be dragging junk along for the ride, both metaphorically and physically. If only my emotions could be sorted through so systematically, but in the meantime, I am still undecided. Should I still have a collection of ransom note magnets on the fridge? At my age?

24th June 2013

Like, Really?

Bless her diamond-encrusted heart. Shortly before her
£7 million wedding, Tamara Ecclestone was sent five pairs
of designer flat shoes by InStyle magazine - totaling £2040
- and 'challenged' (yes, they used that verb) to hang up her
heels and spend a week in flats. Like, OMG.

Tamara informs us that she has hundreds of pairs of
heels. Well, of course. She confesses that when the box of
flats arrived, 'I was worried; to be honest, my heart
sank...they kind of offend me.' Flat shoes offend her? Oh,
to face Tamara's totes tragic challenges.

But for the sake of the article and no doubt the hefty
fee and the chance to promote her new beauty line
available exclusively at Harvey Nichols, she bravely found
a pair she could tolerate and went to dinner. Sadly, she 'felt
really unglamorous and I think people were probably
shocked to see me not in heels.'

Tamara lasted just two days, claiming 'the shoes didn't
make me feel good...I'm definitely not going to buy any.'
Ok then. Sharing the same article, I was expecting more
of Dawn O'Porter, the TV presenter and author who was
flogging her new book, yours for only £7.99. However,
she went to a business meeting in flats 'looking like an
embarrassing auntie. I felt ridiculous. The meeting didn't
go well.' Because of a pair of flats?! What planet, etc, etc.

She rose to the *challenge* though, and soldiered on, despite cheating by wearing a pair of Marc Jacobs' heels on a night out with her husband. The next day she had dinner with her girlfriends, in, gasp, a pair of flats, and splutters, 'I felt like Nora Batty.' One of her friends gleefully told her she looked like her gran.

What can we possibly take away from this insightful piece of investigative journalism? That wearing flats somehow morphs previously vibrant personalities into embarrassing aunties, grans or Nora Batty? Do these outgoing women really need a pair of heels to feel normal? I fear their psyches are more fragile than they would have us believe.

Anyway, before you chuck the flats in the bin, girls, send them my way. I'm a proud member of the Flat Shoe Club (TM) and we didn't really want you as members anyway. So there. I'm also proud to be an embarrassing auntie and am more than happy to be stumbling in flats.

28th June 2013

Stumbling Vs Kettlebell - The Smackdown

After months of staring each other down, I finally decided to pick up my kettlebell, even though it was a very handy doorstop.

On my fridge I have a printout of a nubile, semi-clad, skinny female (not jealous) doing all manner of strange exercises with one of the blasted things and the write up was suitably encouraging - 'kettlebell training is fun and varied, never boring, safe for any age, shape or size.' Not only that, it also promised me 'explosive power.'

Last night, with nothing left to lose except my dignity and a good few pounds, I put down my Walnut Whips and tentatively picked it up. Then swiftly put it back down again and attempted to unscrew two of the weights to make it a tiny bit more manageable.

Exhausted from the effort, I rested long enough to watch the last episode of Mad Men and finish the last Whip before trying again. I hid myself in the kitchen as The Teenager is fond of rushing downstairs yelling out sports results at regular intervals throughout the evening and the humiliation would be too much. Ok, squat and lift. Creakily I lowered myself downwards holding the much-lighter kettlebell. And stopped. Just had to stand up straight again.

My calf muscles, one of which was fully-cramped with MS pain, protested loudly. I down-scaled the reps from 10 to 5, then 3. Next exercise, I just had to swing the thing round my body, switching hands halfway through. Easy. I happily did this for a while, feeling smugly in the rhythm until disaster struck. My dodgy MS hand decided to simply let go. The kettlebell flew towards the cat food bowl, scattering crunchy biscuits across the floor and landed with an almighty thud. Luckily the cat wasn't eating at the time or we'd be holding a memorial service today.

The Teenager rushed downstairs. I stumbled out to stop him in his tracks. 'Muuuuuuum! What's wrong with your face? Why are you all sweaty and red?' 'Oh, you know. Just washing up. So what's the latest score?'

I tried one last exercise. This ball of fear was not going to get the better of me. I raised it above my head, slightly to the left just in case my hand decided to play another joke and I knocked myself unconscious. Not bad. I could feel my muscles stretching. Three reps and I was done.

Amount of exercise? Two and a half minutes. Time spent clearing up the mess and cooling down? Half an hour. Not bad for a first attempt. We will meet again tomorrow, same time, same place.

30th June 2013

Do You Have MS? Take The Quiz!

There's a good reason our neurologists and MS nurses warn us not to google MS. A tweet went round recently with a link to a website that promised to diagnose you with MS or not, just by answering 12 simple questions. I took the quiz, with the knowledge I have already been diagnosed with highly-active relapsing MS.

The website's Androctor Anna, however, gave me unexpected news - 'I screened you for multiple sclerosis. Based on your answers, you don't fit the diagnostic criteria for the screened disease.' I admit, when my neurologist first diagnosed me with Clinically Isolated Syndrome, which may or may not lead to MS, then told me not to look for answers on the internet, the first thing I did when I got home was pour myself a stiff drink, boot up the computer and surf. Endlessly. I'll bet most of you did too.

I can laugh at these quizzes now, but if I had found them back then, would it have been a more serious matter? Would it have reassured me? Through trial and a lot of errors, I eventually stuck to only two websites - The MS Society and the MS Trust. Friends were just as naive as me though - my inbox was flooded with links to various websites. One admonished me for drinking diet Coke, whilst others offered amazing herbal cures or secrets to beating MS, if only I paid hundreds of pounds for the privilege.

More worryingly, other websites chastised me for putting sun cream on my son. By 'denying' him vitamin D, I had unwittingly increased his chances of developing MS. And it's not just internet websites. Have a look at some of the books for sale about beating MS:

- The Hippy Guide to Eliminating Multiple Sclerosis (Sugar Diet Illness)

- Talking Back to MS - How I Beat Multiple Sclerosis Using Low-Dose Naltrexone

- Fighting the Dragon: How I Beat Multiple Sclerosis

I'm sure some of these books have merit, but MS is still an incurable disease. Providing false hope through books, diets or remedies is cruel. MS can be managed, not cured. And are we under pressure to fight back at all costs, rather than concentrate on disease modifying drugs and adjusting to a life with MS?

One thing is certain though, where there is illness, you can be sure there are people out there making money off the back of it.

2nd July 2013

A World Drained of Colour

Part of my job recently has been to source disability aids for a bathroom refurbishment. I rose to the challenge and visited a local showroom. Stepping in from the high street, I entered a grim emporium of bandage-beige and clinical white, an environment utterly devoid of style and colour.

Sun-faded posters depicted happy pensioners looking up at their carers, overjoyed to be using a walk-in bath or grab-rail. There were pictures of sunsets and autumn leaves, the subliminal message all too clear.

This is the medical model of disability in all its soul-sapping starkness. I asked the bored assistant for a fold-up bath chair. She waved a hand vaguely in a direction towards the back of the jumbled shop. One sad little model. White, wall attachments, two legs and a seat. The price for this utilitarian piece of plastic? £85. Someone's having a laugh.

Hesitantly, I interrupted the assistant from her Hello! magazine again to ask what other colours they came in. The blank look on her face was my answer.

Back at home, I searched the internet for modern, fun aids. You've got to look long and hard. I found cool crutches, funky wheelchairs and loads of brilliant walking sticks but struggled to find semi-decent home adaptations.

The heartening message is, visible aids that are seen in public have been updated - crutches, sticks, glasses, wheelchairs (but at a price). At home, however, where most of us probably spend the majority of our time, the manufacturers have helpfully recreated that hospital vibe, as if you need reminding that yes, you are disabled.

Disability aid design is a dusty, neglected area. I'm guessing there's no prizes for designing a toilet chair that could actually put the fun into functional. Perhaps in the shape of a throne, or a racing car? Or stair-lifts that might fitted neatly into a home, rather than looking and sounding like a clunky, depressing piece of functional machinery.

I used to know a young man with a severe disability. He hated having to use a urine bottle at night and told me he wanted one that wasn't so depressing looking - something brightly coloured, or designed to look like a bottle of beer. Something, anything rather than what he had. Not too much to ask?

6th July 2013

Blazing Rows

Our tranquil little cottage has become a battleground, with neither me nor The Teenager willing to give way. There have been tears, sulks and door slamming and I've apologised to the neighbours who rolled their eyes and said, 'Teenagers, eh?' in sympathetic tones.

He's even attempted a hunger strike but lasted only until I stocked the fridge with his favourite Müller yoghurts and waved a pizza under his nose. The cause of all this conflict? His school is adopting a new uniform policy as of September.

From the age of four, The Teenager has gone to school in some variation of a polo top and school jumper. Now his high school want to have a smarter uniform so the kids no longer look like over-grown infants and I'm all for it. We got the final uniform list a couple of days ago and he remains distinctly unimpressed.

'Oh, lovely, you have to wear a blazer!'

'Yeah, with, like, gold piping. I'm not a girl. I'm not wearing it. They can't make me. It's like, rank.'

'But they wear them in Waterloo Road. Very smart.'

'Yeah, whatever. Still not wearing it. It's against my yooman rights'

'Well, look, you get a nice tie as well! Very grown up. Why's it a clip on one though? What's wrong with a proper one?'

'Like, duh, it's so we don't strangle each other. Elf 'n' safety, innit?'

And so we go round in circles. He's trying to organise a boycott for September, but few of his friends are brave/daft enough to join him. The uniform is due to land in the shops within the next couple of weeks and he's coming with me whether he likes it or not.

This may involve an after-school swoop, where I thrust a packet of crisps into his hand, bundle him into the car and lock the doors from the inside. I have tried to reason with him, but as soon as I started a conversation with the words, 'when I was your age....' he huffed and puffed, stomped upstairs and blasted his music out (Oasis, full volume, same two songs in an endless loop).

I will win this argument but the next battle will be trying to take his photograph in his brand new shiny uniform on the first day of Year 10, minus the rude gestures. And there was me thinking the toddler years were the worst.

8ᵗʰ July 2013

Forty Shades of Grey

Here's a quick quiz - just how many signs of ageing are there? Five? Seven? Or, gulp, ten? Step forward Rachel Weisz who was recently flogging 'Revitalist Repair 10', targeting 10 signs of ageing in one overpriced blob of cream.

I'm obviously not at all jealous she's married to Daniel Craig, but I was chuckling when I heard that her TV advert had been banned in the UK after the 'shocking' discovery that she was airbrushed for the advert.

So what are these doom-laden Signs of Ageing and who decides? As I approach the sad day when I will be forced to wear a humorous 'Still Flirty at Forty!' badge to a local restaurant where the chairs will be tied with 'Over the Hill' helium balloons, here's my ten signs of ageing:

1. My mum asks me what I want for this milestone birthday. Without missing a beat I answer ' a super-duper electric toothbrush'.

2. I never, ever sit on the floor, as I would need three strong children to help me up and would probably say 'ooof' a lot.

3. I have a sudden, inexplicable urge to visit garden centres. Not only that, I enjoy a nice cup of tea and a slice of cake in the café afterwards.

4. I read those 'Innovation' catalogues that fall out of the weekend newspapers from cover to cover. And make a list.

5. My colleague has a baby. He is young enough to be my son. Which means I am old enough to be a grandmother.

6. I own not one but two pairs of slippers. Comfy.

7. I talk to my plants. And they talk back. Honestly.

8. I no longer feel it's appropriate to buy Rimmel make-up. Too....bright.

9. I circle TV programmes I want to watch in the Radio Times with a special pen. Antiques Roadshow? Tick.

10. I'm tempted to start listening to The Archers.

I could also say I forget things, I drop things and I have a special non-slip mat in the shower, but I'm blaming all that firmly on the MS.

My plan? To age disgracefully, embarrass The Teenager and start investing in control underwear chic black cashmere jumpers, teamed with lots of large, colourful beads. And start calling everyone 'daahhling' when I can't remember their names...

10ᵗʰ July 2013

Why Is MS So Difficult To Describe?

As if going through the MS diagnostic process isn't difficult enough, trying to describe MS symptoms to the uninitiated is even harder.

Take the MS hug. Cute name, excruciatingly painful. The first time this happened to me, I was in the office. The pain came out of the blue, and as I held my ribs in breathless agony, my colleague politely asked why I was rocking in my chair, making funny gasping noises. After I'd told her it felt like a boa constrictor had wrapped itself round my body, she gave me a curious look and continued typing.

Or the exotically named L'hermitte's sign. Electric shocks in the neck? Maybe it's all in my head. Uhthoff's Phenomenon? Try explaining the torture of frying from the inside out, the complete inability to do anything in the heat. The sadness as you watch the world go by from your window, life happening elsewhere, make-up sliding slowly southwards. Or the tragic look I got from my son the other day when he came home from school to find me with a bag of frozen peas balanced on my head.

Tell anyone else you're heat intolerant (and it's even got a fancy name) and you'll get a barrage of 'Oooooh, me too! Can't stand the heat!' I bore myself silly trying to make them understand it's not just a case of sitting in the shade with a sunhat on, sipping an icy-cold Pimm's. It keeps you locked in the house, limbs trembling, industrial-sized fan on full blast. With our current heatwave, even my head is trembling so much I look like a nodding dog. Or a weeble-wobble.

What about neuropathic pain? The constant buzzing, tingling, throbbing, burning in my feet and legs. It's like having mobile phones strapped to my feet, set to vibrate, with a bit of pincushion-y pain mixed in. Or there's other days when I can't feel my feet at all. But the biggie, as we all know, is the teeth-gnashing frustration of describing MS fatigue.

No matter how you explain it to other people, there will always, always be someone who says, 'Oh, I get tired too. I know exactly what you mean.' Um, no, you don't. Now, please run into my fist. I'm too tired to punch you.

14th July 2013

Guilty As Charged

Something lovely happened yesterday that also broke my heart into tiny pieces.

The Teenager had arranged to go out biking with his friends in the morning. That was great - he's an outdoorsy kid and I'd much rather he was out than stuck in his bedroom in front of the computer screen. He phoned me early afternoon to tell me excitedly he'd been invited to the beach by some of his friends and their parents. When I got home, he was in the middle of packing his swimming costume, a towel and some money, bouncing around, beaming from ear to ear. I waved him off, sat at the kitchen table and cried.

Why? MS. Extreme heat intolerance means I will never be able to take him to the beach in the summer. I can't take him anywhere in this weather. Add constant fatigue on top and I'm a pretty useless parent now.

I'm only glad we did a lot together when he was younger, before MS reared its ugly head. I'm trying to stay positive. The flipside to my new working hours is that I am always at home after school. He might only want to say a few words/grunts before raiding the fridge, but I listen.

I know all the dramas going on at school, I know what homework he needs to hand in and he knows I'm always there for him. Finding a new way of parenting with MS

223

has been one of the hardest challenges and one we are still working out together. Gone are the days we jumped in the car on a whim and headed off. Everything is meticulously planned now, with one eye on the weather forecast and energy levels.

Years ago I was told that when you give birth to a child, you also give birth to a lifetime of guilt. What you feed your child, which toys you buy, which school you send them to - all are guilt-laden. Throw in a hefty dose of MS and the guilt skyrockets.

I'm failing as an active parent. I can only hope that when he looks back as an adult, my son will not remember the times I didn't take him to the beach, but will instead feel secure in the knowledge that he was always, always the centre of my world.

18th July 2013

Scaredy Cat

A couple of days after my last A level, I boarded a train with £90 in my pocket and a one-way ticket to Vienna. With my Doc Martin boots and schoolgirl German, I was ready to take on the world.

Four years later, I went home, courage (or naivety) having taken me to several continents and back, with enough adventures to last a lifetime. These days, I look back at that time with wonder. Who was that person and where is she now?

The other day, someone said to me, 'Oh, you're so brave, the way you cope with MS.' Am I? Thinking about it, no, I'm not brave at all. I'm scared beyond belief. And what's this 'brave' thing all about anyway? Why do people think it's a compliment to tell someone with a life-long illness they're brave? What's the alternative?

One thing I do know, my courage has deserted me. I'm not brave. I'm just making the most of a terrible situation. MS has split my courage right down the middle. Yes, I stood up to bullying at work. Yes, I fought my way through the NHS. On the other hand though, MS symptoms have stripped me of my day to day courage.

I drive as little as possible. I walk as little as possible. I don't go out in the sun. I sleep rather than socialise. Everything is planned right down to the last detail. In short, I am boring. Did I really drink Champagne on a train station roof in Poland for my 20th birthday? Did I really move to New York on a whim? What happened?

After I mentioned this to my mum, she kindly said, 'you haven't lost your courage, it's just been re-directed.' In a way, she is right. MS was a curve-ball that dismantled life as I knew it. Courage didn't come in sweeping gestures, it came bit by bit as I slowly put my life back together.

Tenacity drove me forward and got me through the long, lonely nights when I wept into my wine glass. I'm working on changing from being boring back into a semblance of my former self. So if you see someone drinking Champagne on the roof of Cardiff Central in August, holding an 'I'm 40!' balloon, that'll be me.

22nd July 2013

Wish Me Luck As You Wave Me Goodbye

I'm off to hospital today for my second Campath (Alemtuzumab) infusion and have spent the weekend preparing myself. The Teenager's in London, the house is quiet and my bag is packed.

This year, I'm taking no chances. The first thing to go in the bag were two soft and squishy pillows. Last time around, one of the nurses hunted high and low to provide me with an NHS pillow and came back holding a sad slab of foam.

I've also got my bags of dried fruit and nuts, a family-sized pack of Jelly Babies, some Belvita breakfast bars, a mini hand-held fan, a stack of books (which I probably won't read) and some earplugs.

I've had a lovely, relaxing weekend. On Saturday, my boss took me out for a pre-Campath dinner at a local marina. This is in sharp contrast to last year's Campath treatment, when I was working for a boss who would sack me for having MS just a few months later. There were no good wishes, no cards, no phone call to ask how I was doing. Thankfully, that's all ancient history.

I held a Listeria Feast yesterday, eating all the foods I won't be able to enjoy for three months - salami, sushi, coleslaw, fruit salad, raw carrots and a huge tub of soft serve ice cream. Also some camembert, which I don't even like, but if I'm going to be denied it for three months, I was going to eat it for good measure (nope, still don't like it).

Staying for three days on a neurology ward means that my days will be filled with answering questions from nervous-looking people booked in for lumbar punctures. Hmm, tricky one. If I lie and say it's a breeze, they'll quite possibly drag me out of bed and beat me up afterwards. If I tell the truth, based on my own horrific experience, they'll run screaming from the ward before the needle's even gone near them.

So, wish me luck. Just hoping I can still tweet from my hospital bed...

25th July 2013

Campath 2, Multiple Sclerosis 0

Well, I'm back home from hospital and reunited with my sofa after my second course of Campath.

Having a combination of steroids and Campath over three days has left me exhausted but with a brain that refuses to sleep, so I'm not only a vampire with the continuing heat we're having, but a shuffling, glazed-eyed zombie to boot.

What makes it all worth it though is that I have gone from having relapse after relapse to not having had a single one since my first course last summer. I still have the same symptoms, but there has been no progression - a bit like being frozen in time for a while, giving me breathing space to get my life back into some sort of order.

The hospital stay was brilliant, thanks to amazing staff, superb care and friendly fellow-inmates. One brave patient a few beds down from me let me test drive her swish mobility scooter one evening. Making sure I had the dial set to 'tortoise' speed rather than 'hare', I trundled up the corridor, executed a rather neat three-point-turn and reverse parked the scooter next to her bed again to a modest round of applause. After being hooked up to an infusion for most of the day, the freedom was exhilarating.

The hospital food arrived regular as clockwork and was, well, let's just say, designed to be eaten by people with only a few, if any, teeth left. If I'd been given a straw rather than a knife and fork, I wouldn't have been surprised.

But steroids had given me a ravenous appetite and I ate it all, then ate all the food my mum brought me in afterwards, then woke up starving in the middle of the night and rummaged around in my bedside drawer for biscuits I had stashed away.

Aside from the actual treatment, probably the best thing about the last three days was being in an environment where MS was normal, and nowhere near the most serious illness being treated. It was a relief to chat openly to other patients with no need to explain anything. I think the steroids must have given me not only an uncontrollable appetite, but a bit of a motor mouth too. One patient's regular visitor quipped, 'blimey, it's awfully quiet in here when that Scottish girl reads her book.....'

27th July 2013

Weak As A Kitten

Compared to last year's Campath infusion, I'm a whole lot more tired this time around. Mind you, 'tired' doesn't even begin to describe it - that'd be a bit like saying you're a tad sleepy when in fact you've been poleaxed by MS fatigue. Utterly, thoroughly, totally exhausted would be more apt. Drained of energy, flat battery, squashed, deflated.

Since I got back from hospital on Wednesday afternoon, I have wobbled unsteadily between my sofa, my bed, the fridge and microwave. Right now, these are the four cornerstones of my daily life, with regular medication punctuating the long hours in between.

Alongside all my usual pills, I need to take anti-histamines four times a day for a week and anti-virals twice a day for a month. If I had the energy to jump up and down, I'd rattle. I feel nauseous and spaced out. Thoughts float into my mind and float back out again. The world is either moving a second too slow or a second too fast. I can't work out which. Everything is slightly fuzzy round the edges.

I have little five-minute pockets of energy, when I raise myself from the sofa and slowly stumble around the house finding little jobs to do, just so I feel I'm doing something. Only problem is, I forget halfway through what I was meant to be doing. I stand for minutes, staring at a pair of socks in my hands. What am I supposed to do with them? Or, why am I holding an empty toilet roll?

The steroids don't seem to have left my system quite yet either, so I wake up in the middle of the night and still have a ravenous appetite. I'm like a locust, stripping the food cupboards bare. Half a packet of digestives, circa last year? Yes please. Two bits of dried apricot stuck together? Nom nom.

All this to one side though, I am thankful that at least I know I will feel better very soon, unlike a relapse when it's anyone's guess. There is a definite end in sight.

29th July 2013

Sofa, So Good

The good news is, the steroids I took alongside
Campath have left my system. The bad news is, my sofa is
beginning to take on a Stumbling-shaped dent, so much so
that if the cat dares to jump onto it when I'm not there,
she slides into the dip in the middle. Which is quite funny,
if, like me, you don't get out much.

With the steroids gone, at least I sleep through the
night and no longer wake up at 2 am with a burning desire
to rearrange my herbs and spices into alphabetical order.
All I'm left with now is overwhelming fatigue, but as an
experienced MSer, that's second nature.

The Teenager is back from London. The washing
machine is on, there's thick clouds of Lynx in the
bathroom, food is disappearing from the fridge at an
alarming rate and I'm tripping over his size 12 trainers. All
back to normal.

My plan for this week is a simple one. Sleep, watch
telly, read and repeat. The aim is to a) recover completely
and b) bore myself so silly that I'll be ready for world
domination at the end of it. Or something similar.

My sofa will once again be my command centre. I have
my t.v. listings magazine, the land line, my mobile, the
remote control, a selection of hand creams in case I feel
like doing something energetic. A book, a pile of

magazines, my duvet, the cat, a bag of sweets (or three), and a brochure for the local arts centre. I might not be able to go just yet, but I will absorb some culture by osmosis.

Choice of clothing is also very important. Nothing too tight fitting. The aim is to be comfortable, but also, when I have visitors, I want to look floaty and serene. No slippers (trip hazard and, let's face it, a touch naff). Hair will be washed, as I don't really want the mad woman in the attic look. It's a tiring business, being poorly. Actually, it could be my full time job. Well, at least for a week. After that, I will be back to my normal self. Lazing on the sofa, eating sweets, etc.....

31st July 2013

And This Is What You Could Have Won

A post caught my eye on the MS Society forums the other day. An anonymous person wrote, 'what would you have done if you didn't have MS?'

There were some curt replies - 'a futile question', 'this question is a bit pointless', 'I don't think there's any point wondering about this.' But the second part of the question actually gave it a point - 'Or have you been able to do all the things you want or wanted to do with just a few adjustments?'

I think this is perfectly reasonable to ask, especially as it was posted in the 'new diagnosis and before diagnosis' forum. Isn't this what we all ask ourselves after we've been diagnosed? Someone also replied that this was the same as wondering what it would have been like to be born a boy instead of a girl. Well, no, it isn't. We'd be none the wiser if that had happened.

MS generally strikes in the middle of someone's life, there is a definite before and after. Since being diagnosed, I have had to tweak my career path. Who knows if it's better or worse than what I had previously planned? It's just been modified to take MS into account.

In a twisted way, MS has added a sense of purpose and drive to my life, which, truth be told, was meandering quite merrily towards an unknown destination. Essentially, MS has given me a massive boot right where I needed it. MS made me reconsider my life from every single angle, and how many people get that chance whilst still relatively young?

Or is it just too easy to blame MS for everything? 'It's not me, it's my MS.' It's a cast-iron excuse, something to fall back on when the going gets tough. I hold my hands up. There were many, many times when I wailed 'my life is over, s'over, s'not fair.'

For almost two years I convinced myself I had no future, nothing worthwhile to contribute to society. But if we have to live with MS, we have to make it work for us. So, if we look at the question again, we could ask ourselves, 'What would you have done if you didn't have MS, and why aren't you doing it?'

2nd August 2013

Busy Doing Nothing

I've had a very productive week doing very little except recovering from Campath. You need to put in a lot of preparation work to do nothing.

First up, food. I've spent hours on the computer putting together a shopping list for Ocado home delivery to save me the hassle of going to the shops. With a brain functioning at less than zero, it was a Herculean task. I also Blame The Brain(TM) for the abundance of snacks and chocolate that found their way into my virtual basket and the lack of proper, grown-up things such as leafy green vegetables and washing up liquid.

Next, The Teenager. Unlike me, he's had a busy week doing an awful lot and needs frequent cash injections and food (see above point). He's also keeping me 'entertained' with a detailed breakdown and analysis of the upcoming football season, so I've had to try and concentrate as he throws in random pop quizzes to check I've been listening.

Then there's the cat. She also wants feeding. On Tuesday, her Go-Cat crunchy biscuits didn't quite fill the gap so she brought in a barely-alive bird and dropped it at my feet. I screamed, she ran away with the poor thing and proceeded to eat it, head first, outside my window, casting me triumphant glances as she munched away.

I am also not studying, not doing any housework, not getting rid of the cobwebs (18 and counting, plus two large, dead spiders spinning around, eww). I am busy lolling on my sofa, reading trashy magazines and watching trashy telly. This keeps me occupied for hours and hours, leaving no time to just do nothing.

To break the monotony, I went with the boss to Ikea the other day to look at kitchens. I've never been one to turn down free meatballs. I did nothing much at Ikea either but on my way through the Market Hall, I picked up a lamp I didn't really need. Ikea does strange things to the mind. It's virtually impossible to leave without buying anything, even if it's just a 60p hotdog or a dustpan and brush set. So that's been my week.

Next week I'm planning to do more of the same. It might look like I'm doing nothing but I'm rushed off my feet.

6th August 2013

My MS Is Worse Than Your MS

For me, the best side effect of having MS is the support of fellow MSers. MS nurses, neurologists, charities are brilliant, but there's nothing like talking to another person with MS. They just....understand. Whether they're virtual friends made on Twitter and through blogging or people I've got to know in person over the past few years, the support is incredible. No worry is too small to share, no question too random.

So why is there an insidious underbelly of hierarchy among people with MS? When did MS become a competition? I have heard many variations on these comments:

- 'You've only got relapsing remitting? Hah! You don't know the half of it.'

- 'Oh, I've been in a wheelchair for years, you don't know how fortunate you are.'

- 'How many times a day do you fall over/trip/stumble?'

- 'You're lucky, there's nothing they can do for me. I just suffer with it.'

- 'Wish *I* could be in remission, I just get worse and worse.'

239

- 'Are you *sure* you've got MS?'

And the absolute killer when it comes from someone with MS, 'But you look so WELL.'

I'm glad to say these people are in the minority, but it still cuts deep. Should I not be allowed to say I'm in remission for fear of upsetting other people? Shouldn't we be celebrating new advances in disease modifying drugs rather than sneering at those who have the opportunity to take them?

Then there are those people for whom MS becomes their entire raison d'être. They exist in an MS bubble, proud of their suffering status. They are unwilling to say or do anything that's not connected to the huge cross they bear. And more often than not, these people aren't even the worst affected by MS.

Whilst it is comforting to be surrounded by fellow MSers, this does not define my life, just as MS doesn't. I may have to live with MS but it certainly isn't the focal point of everything I do. That would be as good as giving up. For me, it is far more positive to show that you can live a rewarding and fulfilling life alongside MS.

We might not be able to cure MS just yet, but we can begin by dropping the competitive element. Aren't we all in it together?

8th August 2013

This Is What MS Feels Like

Imagine you had a life-long friend. This friend's been with you through everything. Every high, every low. Seen you through weird and wonderful adventures across the world, the birth of your child, a near-fatal car crash.

One day, this friend turns on you. To begin with, you don't really take much notice, you're too busy trying to get on with life. You ignore the niggling doubts. You trust this friend implicitly, with your life. But the warning signs become hard to ignore.

You're sure they're drugging your coffee, it's the only explanation for the overwhelming fatigue. They begin messing with your mind, mixing up your thoughts, your emotions, garbling your speech. Things escalate badly. They begin pushing you over and tripping you up. You never know when it's going to happen and you start to live in fear. Your balance is shot to pieces, the pain is uncontrollable. You start going out less, hiding yourself at home.

You're bullied at work because of the friend, who by now is an enemy. This will ultimately be an excuse to fire you from a job you love. Friends abandon you, leaving you even more isolated. Your family can't begin to understand what's happening to you, no matter how many times you try to explain. Your income drops as you have to reorganise your working hours, your social life is non-existent.

Simple tasks become mountains you have no hope of scaling. Just getting through each day in one piece becomes your sole aim. Fear and loneliness are now your constant companions, keeping you up into the small hours, frantically working out what your new future will look like, if you have one at all.

Every area of your life is rapidly changing beyond recognition, so fast you can barely keep up. Your son cries in his bedroom. He can't cope and you don't know quite how to console him when you can't even reassure yourself. This is what MS feels like.

Your body, your friend through life who has never let you down before, attacks you from every single angle. Drugs, treatments and a superb support network have restored some kind of order to my life, although it is not the life I had before. But those black, dark days will remain with me forever. And they may, just may, reappear at any time. Carpe diem.

12th August 2013

That Was The Decade That Was

On the eve of my foray into my forties, I'm indulging myself by looking back on the last decade.

This time ten years ago, I had no real idea which direction my life was taking. My twenties had been a whirlwind of travelling, angsty, late-night discussions in dark cellar bars, falling in and out of love and The Teenager (The Baby?) who made a late, messy and noisy arrival eight days after I turned 26.

I swapped crisp white shirts and hours spent lingering over black coffee and Gitanes for years of finger-painting, wet wipes and traipsing round the local parks. At 32, after four years of study, I qualified as a homeopath. My clinic took off and I adored my work until the recession brought it to a sudden halt.

I switched my attention to a degree course in health and social care, laying careful plans for the future. The years passed. Endless sleepovers, fish fingers, day trips, gold star stickers, football magazines and scooters. Rugby kits and shoes got bigger and dirtier each year, those tiny baby slippers a 'was he ever that small?' distant memory.

As he got older, I could even have friends over for girlie nights in without the fear of a near-naked child hurtling at top speed down the stairs, entirely decorated in felt-tip pen and a Superman cape. And now he's suddenly a full-blown Teenager. All six foot of him. I adore him, even when he grunts and holds his hand out for yet more money.

MS dominated my late thirties, turned everything upside down and we're still picking our way through the aftermath. Career plans have changed as have priorities. MS certainly isn't the best method for working out what's important in life, but it's helped. Everything is more in focus now and I take nothing for granted.

So how were my thirties? Probably the decade where life shifted on its axis. The dreams and expectations I had at the start of them are long-gone. In its place is the realisation is that anything is possible. I just need to get out there and make it happen.

14ᵗʰ August 2013

Business As Usual

Well there goes another birthday and I have now well
and truly entered my fifth decade. The candles on my cake
took an embarrassingly long time to blow out even with
the help of The Teenager, fire extinguisher at the ready just
in case. I was half-expecting the Birthday Fairy to present
me with wisdom and maturity befitting my advanced years,
but sadly it seems I'm off her list for now.

The Teenager had promised to set his alarm for 6.30
and make me breakfast in bed (probably a pot of yoghurt
and a glass of milk - he seems incapable of working the
toaster or kettle), but by 8 I shook him awake, starving and
eager to open my birthday cards.

My mantle-piece is now festooned with helpful
reminders of my age, just in case MS cog fog made me
forget. As my official Big Birthday Bash isn't till the end
of the month, I spent the evening indulging myself in a 5-
step 'youth-boosting' home facial. This included
exfoliation, a time reversal face mask, firming youth serum,
a lift and brighten eye complex (complex? Huh?) and
finally a-stop-the clock moisturiser. The instructions
suggested that 'for the ultimate spa experience, light a
fragranced candle and have some gentle music playing'.

I didn't have a scented candle, so I sprayed lavender air
freshener around and instead of music, The Teenager was
watching the Ashes highlights up loud. After I had applied

the final blob of moisturiser, I rushed to the mirror,
hoping to see all 58 signs of ageing erased and a 20-year
old version of myself staring back at me. Disappointment
is below an understatement. Instead of baby-soft skin, I
was greeted with a bright red face punctuated by two dots
where my eyes normally are. Sigh.

To help me over the shock, I had a third slice of
birthday cake and a(nother) cheeky glass of wine. I always
expect significant birthdays to be like New Year's Eve. At
the stroke of midnight, I will be magically transformed into
a brand-new, shiny person, leaving the baggage of the
previous years behind me, like a rom-com film made real.
That didn't happen, so I waited 'til 8.04pm, the time I was
actually born (spinning it out, yup). And? Nope, nothing.
I'm still the same old me.

16th August 2012

Fight Back Or Be Damned

One of my pet hates is people with chronic illnesses being urged to 'fight back' by others who have no idea what they're talking about. Am I supposed to feel better when someone looks at me with sad eyes, grasps my hand and tells me, 'oh, you're so brave, I just know you can fight this thing.'

Perhaps the media is partly to blame, when every third-rate 'celebrity' who is diagnosed with anything is featured in trashy magazines claiming they will fight back, not let it beat them, blah, blah, blah. Ironically, they usually end their not-so-exclusive interview with a coy plea for privacy.

How exactly am I supposed to fight back against MS? It isn't going to go away. Oh sure, I could pay thousands for quack cures, immerse myself in healing waters, start meditating, follow a Beat MS Diet, howl at the moon. And yes, I probably would feel slightly better, just as anyone without MS would also feel slightly better following a strict, healthy regime.

Isn't it better for us to adapt to our new lives with MS rather than fighting the unfightable? It's not about giving in to it, it's about getting on with it. There is a creeping sense of a hidden agenda embedded within this call to fight back. Anyone with an illness must resist being 'different' at all costs. We must strive to regain our 'normality', that which is acceptable to mainstream society.

We must fight back against anything that marks us as being outside the socially acceptable norm and if we appear not to be fighting back, then we're obviously not trying hard enough.

How often do we hear, 'Oh, she fought a brave battle' or 'she just gave up the fight.' This kind of pressure only makes life with MS more difficult than it already is. The only thing I'm fighting back against is the discrimination that comes with having MS. Being sacked from work because of it. Struggling to find a new job because of it. The constant blank, disbelieving faces when I try and fail to describe overwhelming fatigue and the reality of living with a mostly invisible illness.

In the meantime, I'm sticking with Jack Osbourne's philosophy - Adapt and Overcome. Interestingly, it's his family who talk about fighting back, not him. Anyone who wants to make me feel guilty for not fighting back hard enough, stumble for a week in my shoes, then come and talk to me.

18th August 2013

Any Time, Any Place

If they gave out medals for sleeping, I'd be top of the podium (after a quick nap). I wake up tired, I go to bed tired. I yawn constantly. And not polite little yawns either. Massive, jaw-aching, cartoon-like yawns. 'Am I boring you?' is a phrase I hear an awful lot.

It's exhausting (excuse the pun) being tired all the time. It's a bit like MS in miniature - the feeling of being disconnected from society, in a little bubble all of my own. Days are meticulously planned, pockets of time doled out like bargaining chips.

There is a famous spoon theory, to explain chronic tiredness to other people, about how you only have a set amount of energy in one day. I prefer to think of the Mallet Theory. Say you start the day with ten mallets. You have to give one up every time you feel you've been coshed over the head by MS fatigue. If you've got any left at the end of the day, it's been a good one.

The thing about MS fatigue, like most other MS symptoms, is that it can be managed, not cured. I have loads of strategies - a handy duvet tucked behind the sofa, rushing around like a wild woman when I suddenly find myself with some precious energy, preparing food ready for later, a command table set up next to my sofa with everything to hand.

In fact, it's very similar to when The Teenager was a screaming cute little baby. The midwife would chastise me, 'now dear, mummy must sleep when baby does, mummy must be guided by baby, baby won't mind if you haven't managed to dust the house.' Baby won't mind if I shut the door on you, then.

I'd like to say I feel better with all this sleep. I don't. It's not a luxury, it's a necessity. It barely brings me back up to my baseline energy levels, and even that's way below par. But as with everything else that MS throws at me, I've adapted to it. It's kind of normal now. Only problem is, I keep running out of mallets.

20th August 2013

Basically, MS Is Crap

I've had a lot of good and a little bit of not-so-good feedback about my recent blog posts. Some people told me in no uncertain terms, 'Oi, you, stop joking about MS, how dare you? And are you not grateful/bowing down/prostrating yourself for all those who are fighting on your behalf, and if you aren't, why the hell not? Sadly, most of these comments were sent to me privately so I'm unable to share them with you.

I have never, ever joked about anybody fighting to find a cure for MS. They are all amazing people doing an incredible job. The only exception is fundraising by fire-walking. Personally, I still find it awfully strange when one of the most common symptoms of MS is heat intolerance. It just seems kind of.....bizarre?

When MS decided to strike for a second time in our family, I cried, ranted and raved and eventually picked myself back up again. I will be forever grateful for advances in medicine which allowed me to choose Campath, a choice my dad never had back in the 1970s. He was simply sent home with a walking stick and told to get on with it. He died when I was four, and the precious few memories I have of him are fragmented.

Why do I joke about MS? I think we all know MS is serious. We live with it day in, day out. So what's wrong with a little light relief? Also, I joke about myself and my symptoms, no one else's. That just wouldn't be funny. Frankie Boyle, please take note.

I just don't understand people who think I should live a serious life just because I have a serious illness. Or is this yet another example of 'disabled' people having to conform to a rigid set of societal expectations? I've cried enough over MS for now. It's here, life has changed and I've changed with it. Like a lot of you, I no longer take things for granted and my life is in much sharper perspective than before. MS is a daily reminder of the fragility of life.

So, yes, MS is crap. It's awful. Regular readers of my blog will know I address this in serious and more light-hearted posts. And I hope my little blog can bring a smile or make someone think, 'yup, me too.'

27th August 2013

Groundhog Day

I was away at the weekend with The Teenager and a friend, who came with me only on the condition that he could watch Formula 1 (yawn).

To pass the ho-hum time away, I read the newspapers and amused myself by reading bits out to him as he tried to concentrate on men in leather onesies going round and round and round in little cars.

'I didn't know Richard Pryor had MS, did you?'

'Nope. Shhh. They're on the 27th lap.'

'Bored.'

'Shhh. Anyway, you've got MS, what's the big deal?'

Of course. I completely forgot I had MS. Weird. I'd like to say it's because I'm in rude health, but it's probably more likely that all my symptoms have now been fully assimilated into my life and it's just...normal?

This happens most days and it's like a short, sharp shock every single time I remember. A bit like mornings when The Teenager was a new-born and it'd dawn on me that I was A Mother. I'd lie there, waiting for him to start yelling (never took long) and wonder why on earth the maternity unit actually let me leave the hospital with him.

When they told me I was free to leave, I looked at the baby then back at them, asking, 'seriously? He's so....um, so, kind of small?' 'Yes love, babies generally are. Now, be a dear and shut the door behind you.'

Will this groundhog day ever end? Of course I know I have MS. My legs, arms and brain tell me. Or is this actually a good thing? Have I come to a point of quiet acceptance?

I mean, I still chuckle when I realise I'm a mother to a teenager. Me? Really? I feel like I was one myself only a few years ago. Or as The Teenager says, 'mum, if you say 'totes' one more time and keep reading Heat magazine, I'll get you a subscription to Women's Weekly for your Christmas.'

30th August 2013

At First I Was Afraid, I Was Petrified

On Wednesday, I had an appointment with my MS nurse to discuss how the latest round of Campath had gone. I had a good chat, did a blood test, made a new appointment for next February and left, happy and relaxed. I'd reached a significant milestone.

This was probably the first MS appointment where the staff haven't had to virtually prise my fingers from the reception desk and tell me to go home, everything will be fine. I always had just one more question, one more point to raise. I could quite happily have set up camp in the waiting room.

At my very first appointment with the neurologist, I left confused and with a head full of unfamiliar medical terminology, stunned that something so potentially huge could be on the horizon. I wanted to stay in that room forever, boring him to tears as I struggled to make sense of what he was telling me.

At appointments with the MS nurses, there was a sense of comfort and safety as I sat in their room, emotions never far from the surface. Having been thrust into an unfamiliar environment, I very quickly didn't want to leave. The MS team had an answer to everything. If I could have taken an MS nurse home, I would have.

The whole MS diagnostic process probably doesn't help. Who knew it can take so long? Who, outside of the MS world has an idea what the McDonald criteria is, what oligoclonal bands are? Not only that, there is the sense that your own world will never be the same. How do you tell your family? How can you cope once you start being bullied at work due to your diagnosis? How bad was my health going to get?

The MS team helped me through it all. I was given access to a vast array of support, equipping me to become my own expert of my MS. It's been a long two years. When I look back to those frightening early days, I marvel at how far I have come. I'm still me, I just happen to have MS, and I now know exactly how to live with it.

7th September 2013

Saved By The Bell

This has been a sad, sad week. The Teenager went back to school on Wednesday and I'm still wiping away the tears, getting used to rattling around an empty house with only Jeremy Kyle for company. There is so much I will miss:

•The feeling of lightness in my wallet. It will take a bit of adjusting to not having to dig deep every single day. Money for the cinema and lunch in town with friends for him, beans on toast and 'Cash in the Attic' with the cat for me.

•Telling the Teenager for the umpteenth time, 'In my day, we ... (insert one of the following - 'didn't have the internet', 'made our own fun out of tin cans and bits of string', 'walked everywhere').

•The loud music blasting from his bedroom when I'm trying to have a quick shut-eye. Everything from Nirvana to the Beach Boys to new stuff I'm far too old to know the names of. He's nothing if not eclectic.

•The drama involved in buying a new school uniform. Will particularly miss the slammed bedroom doors, followed by shouts of 's'not fair, hate school, stoopid Harry Potter blazer.'

•Ditto School Shoe Shopping . I'm sure the lovely lady who helped us really didn't mind bringing out so many boxes of shoes to a Kevin the Teenager lookalike. She did look awfully happy/relieved when we left though.

•The friends who pop over to see The Teenager for an hour and end up staying all day. Such dear, funny little people. Not at all loud.

•The chainsaw snores from The Teenager's bedroom as he has yet another lie-in.

So, forgive me if I'm a touch emotional. I have dug out all the old photographs of his first day at school, stretching back years. They range from the impossibly cute, smiley 4 year old to the one last year, where I had to bribe him with an extra quid for lunch. He's slouched, unsmiling, barely looking at the camera. Sigh.

This year, in his smart new blazer, his photo was more like a mugshot for junior Crimewatch. Anyway, I have to pull myself together and not feel too despondent. As The Teenager couldn't wait to tell me yesterday, it's only six weeks to half-term. Like, yay.

13th September 2013

Things Ain't What They Used To Be

For the last two years I seem to have been lying low, coping with everything MS had to throw at me. I didn't realise just how much the parameters of my life had altered until I went to London on Monday.

I wasn't particularly worried beforehand - I'd lived and studied there for a couple of years, I loved the buzz, the people, the sheer energy the city pulsed with. So I trotted off, took my seat on the train and prepared to reignite my passion for the city.

The first inkling things weren't quite the same as before happened seconds after disembarking at Paddington. Where had all these people come from? Oi, why did you just barge in to me? Where did I put my ticket? Help.

I was swept along by an unforgiving tide of people to the tube station, buffeted from all sides, whimpering, with panic levels going through the roof. What was wrong with me? I used to do the exact same journey with a howling baby, pram and suitcase in tow.

My legs had turned to jelly, my face was bright red with stress and heat as I tried to quell the rising anxiety. I collapsed on to a seat in the tube train, a chattering bunch of Italians clutching maps and water bottles swaying into me every couple of seconds. After my meeting I did the reverse journey in the same dishevelled state. I needed to get home. By teleportation if possible. Or helicopter.

Over lunch before getting back on the Cardiff train, I discussed this with my friend. 'I don't understand!' I wailed, picking at my fish and chips in a ye olde English pub. Had I really changed that much? Out of my five-mile radius comfort zone, it appeared I had. Gone was my fearlessness and energy. I knew my energy levels weren't the same as before, but had they really plummeted so low?

Finally, I made it home. I was a mess. Every nerve was trembling, I was exhausted and mentally shattered. It took me a whole day off work to recover, where I hid at home, coming to terms with what had happened. Reality smacking me right in the face. I'm shocked. I knew things were bad, just not that bad.

15th September 2013

What Are The Chances?

It's never going to be good news when your MS nurse phones up out of the blue and says, 'can you talk?'

To cut a long, uncertain story short, it seems I may, just may, have developed thyroid problems since taking Campath. It's treatable, I'm not too worried and as always, the MS nurse was calm and reassuring. I took the risk, I knew the chances - a 10-30% possibility with Campath, and I have no regrets having had the opportunity to take it.

It has given me my life back. What's frustrating is that I was pretty much signed off by my neurologist until next February and was finally beginning to put the uncertainty of living with MS behind me. Now there's another round of blood tests on top of the monthly Campath one and I'll have an appointment with yet another consultant, an endocrinologist this time.

And what's really, really annoying, is that I seem to have come up with the dodgy odds again. Apparently there's a 1 in 750 chance of developing MS in the first place. Not too bad. If you have a parent with MS as I did, there's around a 1 in 100 chance. That'll be me then. And now with the thyroid odds, I'm beginning to wonder if I'm ever so slightly jinxed.

On the flip side, I'm grateful a potential problem has been picked up so early, and at least I'm already learning to live with some of the symptoms as they're remarkably similar to MS - fatigue, hand tremors, heat intolerance.

I'm wondering though, if you have both MS and thyroid problems, does that mean you get twice the amount of fatigue? And hand tremors? I'm only asking as I'm beyond shattered right now and I broke my second-last glass a couple of days ago, of a brand-new set of four. I have now reluctantly invested in plastic ones. Still drop the blasted things though, but at least they bounce.

Anyway, with the odds stacked in my favour, I'm toying with the idea of taking up scratch cards as a hobby. Or bingo?

17th September 2013

MSpreneurs

Remember that divisive phrase coined to describe mums who create new businesses or turn their hobby into something more serious after giving birth - mumpreneurs? (What happened to dadpreneurs, eh?).

Anyway, I was thinking about this the other day when I was talking to a friend about how much I love writing but never did anything serious about it until MS. Something about a life-altering experience finally giving me a much-needed boot in the right direction.

I have countless pretentious interesting novel ideas floating around, one of which would of course win the next Man Booker Prize if only I could get round to writing more than the title and dedication page. Well, ok, perhaps not, but you get my drift.

When I was younger and living in Europe, I quite fancied myself as a chicly-impoverished author, haunting dark smoky cafés, being invited to literary salons to wax lyrical upon deep, meaningful subjects. So perhaps, just as mumpreneurs are spurred on after their lives have changed, so some of us with MS feel the same?

I've heard from loads of people over the last year - inspiring stories about how you changed jobs or turned a hobby into a satisfying career after being diagnosed with MS. So I have coined a new phrase of my own -

MSpreneur. I quite like the sound of that. It's positive - taking something good out of something so potentially disruptive.

After years of stop-start writing projects, it's been incredible to indulge my passion for writing. This time last year, I sat down with a beginner's guide to Wordpress and blogging. After throwing the book against the wall a few times, I finally worked out how to publish my first post.

Obviously I haven't made a career out of it but MS has, amazingly, thrown up something positive out of the whole terrible process. I'm now off to a dark, non-smoky café. I will nurse my Americano for hours, deep in thought, scribbling notes for a blockbuster. More likely though, it will be my weekly shopping list. Must not forget the loo roll this time.

19th September 2013

Wardrobe Malfunction

So the great news is I've been shortlisted for an MS Society Award and the ceremony will be held at The Dorchester in October. The bad news is the ceremony will be held at The Dorchester in October.

October! Four weeks today to be precise. I've been googling 'Drop A Tonne of Weight in 28 Days', but short of swallowing a tapeworm, I've resigned myself to looking more like Bella Emberg from the Roly Polys than Cara Delevingne's frumpy cousin. Steroids, fatigue and a complete sense of inertia have conspired to pack on the weight over the last two years.

I hold my hands up (hang on, let me just put my Cheezy Puffs down), it's my fault too. When your whole world is falling apart, what's a box or two of Maltesers going to add to it? And that lovely creamy Greek yoghurt with added honey just sweetens the bitter pill. The phrase 'I have nothing to wear' has never been more apt.

Problem number one - flat shoes - how to look suitably glamorous in them? Even if I could squeeze myself into a beguiling little cocktail number, surely the effect would be ruined without even a tiny heel?

A friend helpfully suggested I should forget all about wearing a dress and choose a smart trouser suit instead. And invest in a head-to-toe Spanx bodysuit. And have one of those miracle weight-loss treatments three hours before, where you get wrapped up in cling-film and covered in towels. Hmm. I would quite possibly faint from MS heat intolerance and spend the ceremony lying comatose across three chairs in the nearest A&E.

Problem number two - how to look glam in a trouser suit without looking like I'm going to a job interview?

Problem number three - how to not stumble/drop food down myself/smash a glass during the event. Do you think they'd mind if I took one of my plastic wine glasses along? And a bib? You can see why I'm a bit worried.

And not only that, when I asked The Teenager what he'd be wearing, he mumbled, 'hoodie, innit, but don't stress, I'll wear my smart trainers'. Ye gods.

23rd September 2013

Blood, Sweat And No Ideas

In a little over two weeks, I'll be sitting what I hope will be my final ever exam. A three hour written paper. Having the attention span of a gnat is proving problematic though.

I've spent hours (days, weeks) creating the most fabulous study notes. Colour-coded, bullet-pointed, succinct. They really are quite lovely. I settle myself down, ready to commit some facts to memory. And that's the problem. My memory has taken a long sabbatical and I've got no idea when it's coming back. I read a few study points and my brain is full.

Maybe I'll just rest my eyes for five minutes. An hour later, I wake up with a start, study notes still clutched in my hands. All hope of absorbing essential nuggets of knowledge by osmosis fades. I look over past exam papers with a growing sense of horror. What hope do I have of writing dazzling answers when I can't even understand the questions?

I had such high hopes when I started the university course six years ago. I whizzed through the first four years, feeling smug when I achieved pretty decent essay and exam scores. This was part of my Plan - a new career path which would grow alongside The Teenager, so come graduation, I would be ready for the next stage, an MA.

Then, when The Teenager reached 16, I would step in to a wonderful new job.

Thanks to MS, those dreams now lie in tatters, and my so-called career path has become overgrown and inaccessible. But, hey, I've never been one to give up that easily. I'll do something completely different. Just not quite sure what yet. A non-stressful job that utilises all my talents? I'm thinking cake tester (nah, not enough chocolate in that one, I'll try the other one, ta very much) or a flat shoe expert, where I can try out the very latest styles and give them a thumbs up or down and keep the ones I like.

In the meantime, exam day is fast approaching and my brain is melting under the pressure. I daydream about what life will be like after 1pm on October 9th. I will be free! I will ceremoniously burn all my study notes and raise a toast to the last six years. Despite everything, I will have made it through.

27th September 2013

My Boss, He's Brave

My poor boss, who's been employing me since I was sacked from my last job for having MS, is a very patient man.

He runs his own construction company, so finding a suitable post for me was never going to be easy. I'm very good at my job though - I'm brilliant at helping him out ('you missed a bit, no not there, *there*'), I don't mind eating bacon rolls for breakfast and although he casts longing glances at his radio, I'm sure he much prefers listening to me chattering away about something and nothing in between checking Twitter on my phone and sitting in the van to keep warm.

Thankfully for him, I'm not on site much. More often than not I get to sit at home and make phone-calls and undertake important research, a project manager kind of role. 'Hello, is that Bricking It Ltd?' 'Great, um, I just wondered how much your red bricks are?' 'How many? Oh, that's a good question.' 'Shall we say, enough for an extension? Nope, don't know the size, but it's kind of big.'

Anyway, the Boss decided to have a Quiet Word last week and started with, 'look, this isn't working out, is it?' Oh. As I was about to hand over my Stanley knife, woolly hat and McDonalds coffee loyalty card (only one coffee bean sticker left to collect), he put an interesting proposition to me.

He asked me not only continue to work on his quotes and paperwork, but also keep his website up to date and run a Twitter account in his company name - become his Social Media Manager (posh).

Getting all excited, I grabbed his arm and said, 'Yes! Right, we need to find your voice, sweetie, your voice. What kind of Twitter voice do you want to have? Funny? Factual? Serious?' To cut a long story short (let's just say the Boss's eyes glazed over), he's going to leave that all to me.

Well, my mind's been working overtime. I will tweet the latest Gregg's sausage roll deals, interesting facts about architraves and skirting boards and throw in a few philosophical musings, such as 'the journey of a thousand miles begins with one brick.' I reckon the Boss will be most impressed.

29th September 2013

A Day Off From MS

Last night, after being woken in the wee small hours yet again with nerve pain and unable to get back to sleep, my mind wandered. Just what would it be like to have one full day off from MS? How amazing would that be?

I would spring out of bed, full of beans and head straight for a boiling hot bath, using up my dusty bottle of Matey bubbles. No non-slip bath mat today, no pesky heat intolerance. After a long soak, I'd deftly apply my make-up, managing to execute a perfect sweep of eyeliner.

I'd get dressed easily, no fumbling over buttons, no tripping over my feet and I'd be able to wear jeans I haven't fitted in over two years. And heels! Beautiful heels. How I've missed you. I'd put them on and not take them off all day. I would sashay everywhere. I would stride, head held high. No looking at the pavements.

In fact, I'd take the day off work and spend it walking. Just walking, even in heels. And I'd go to cute little gift shops where I'd be unafraid of picking up glass ornaments or bumping into things or small children.

I'd find a really hot, really busy café and spend a stress-free hour sipping a coffee, people-watching. I'd call up friends out of the blue, suggesting a night out later. I'd know for sure I'd still have the energy. On the way home I'd do all my Christmas shopping in one go, undaunted by the crowds, balancing the bags easily, going through my long list from memory.

Back home, I'd wrap and label all the gifts then cook a fiendishly complex recipe from scratch. I'd spring clean my entire house. I'd even dig out the feather duster. Then I'd do a whole pile of ironing. And spend a couple of hours weeding the garden, all before slipping in to something fabulous (with my heels, natch) and get ready to go out. The evening would pass in a happy blur of catching up with long-neglected friends.

I'd charm them with my wit and fast responses. I'd remember the punchlines to long jokes, I'd carry five drinks at a time back from the bar. I wouldn't come back til gone midnight, falling happily in to bed. Then I'd wake in the wee small hours. With nerve pain.

3rd October 2013

Shops 'n' Strops

Earlier this week, I spent a frustrating couple of hours in the men's changing room at Hollister. There were fumbles, anguished cries and yelling. Yup, I was clothes shopping with The Teenager.

He's at that fussy stage (when isn't he?) - his clothes have to fit just so, the colour has to be just right. Although how he could see anything in Hollister is beyond me. Maybe it's my age, but it's pretty darned gloomy in there. And there's far too many über-handsome staff with chiselled jaws and their underwear on show. Tsk.

After rummaging round in the dark and messing up all the lovely neat displays, The Teenager pulled out a couple of shirts to try on. An hour later (and after profuse apologies to Mr Handsome for all the noise), he emerged from his cubicle and posed before the mirror, turning this way and that, arms flapping.

'Oh, it's a lovely colour! Suits your eyes. Let's buy it.' (looks at watch) 'Nah, it's, like, dunno.'

'What about the other one? Or that one? Or the one you flung across the room?'

'S'not dench, innit?' (Dench? Huh?)

We left empty-handed and repeated the same scenario in the next store. And the next. Normally on trips like this, we have a little family tradition of rounding off the whole drama by taking it in turns to choose a restaurant for dinner. It was my turn.

More eye-rolling and dramatic sighs when I told him I wanted to try a nice, eclectic place he hadn't been to before. 'Wanna go to Nando's. Wanna go to Nando's. Wanna go.....' 'Oi, it's my choice. You'll like it. ' 'My friend said it was a girly place. Wanna go to...' 'How can a restaurant be girly? It's dench!' 'Mum, that's just tragic. Please don't.'

We sat ourselves down in my choice of place, The Teenager grudgingly admitting it wasn't that bad and he admired his new rugby socks (our only purchase), before tweeting his friends a picture of them. Then he facebooked a picture of his burger. We had a lovely meal. Me, The Teenager and his phone. Dench...

9th October 2013

I'm Well Adjusted

My chiropractor called me the other day and said, 'Oi, your boss has just been in for an appointment and told me you don't want to book in as you think you're too fat. Don't be daft, come in!' 'Can't. Too fat. Could break your bench, honestly. Potentially very, very embarrassing.'

I've been visiting the chiropractor for over 12 years now. He magically sorted out my neck problems, brought on by exiting a car through the roof at high speed (not classy, pretty painful) and he's also treated The Teenager since he was a toddler.

That Fateful Day two years ago when I woke up unable to speak or walk properly, he was the first person I called. After talking gibberish, he summoned me to his clinic, ran through some neurological tests and quietly told me to go straight to hospital. He was the first to put MS on the table and helped keep me sane through the long, anxiety-ridden diagnostic process.

Anyway, I went to the clinic, putting all fears of rolling off the bench with an ungainly thud to one side. Thankfully, the chiropractor is a consummate professional and put me at ease straight away as I brought him up to speed with everything that had happened since I last saw him (the list was long and he was awfully patient).

Then it was time to have the treatment. I pulled off my boots with an unladylike 'Oof' and popped (heaved) myself on to the bench. On my front. On my back. On my side. Probably the most exercise I've had in a while. Turn neck this way and that. Leg up, arm down. Why do I always imagine those mice from 'Bagpuss' when I'm lying there? You know, the ones that sing 'we will fix it, we will make it new, new, new?' Marginally better than 'The Flumps' I guess.

I felt like a new woman after the treatment and mentally kicked myself for leaving it so long. My body felt unfurled, stronger. There's not an awful lot that can be done to make living with MS easier, but having regular chiropractic sessions certainly helps. It's like a great big sigh of relief running through my whole body.

Finally, I stood up and asked, 'Lovely! Am I normal now?' With good grace, the chiropractor declined to answer.

11th October 2013

Free At Last

The books have been packed up, the paperwork has been shredded and my house has been cleared of post-it notes and last-minute scribbles. I sat my last ever university exam on Wednesday and it's all over bar the marking.

I nearly gave up after five years, but quite fancied the (Hons) after my name so ploughed on for a final year. It was worth it though and the sense of achievement has been incredible, as was the bottle of bubbly I had waiting in the fridge.

I've been lucky. My MS nurse has written a letter in my defence, something along the lines of, '...please excuse Stumbling, her cat ate her study notes and her brain doesn't work properly'. Which is just as well. I struggle to remember my shopping list, so how on earth was I supposed to remember a whole year's worth of facts, ready to regurgitate onto blank paper? In my shaky handwriting?

It didn't help when a fellow student emailed me the day before asking if I had revised Esping Anderson. If I knew what it/he/she was, perhaps I might have. As it was, to me it just sounded like an Ikea dining table.

Anyway, I arrived at the exam centre, ignored the last minute swotters, and took my seat. I set out my pens and bottle of water. The woman next to me set out a lucky teddy, three bottles of water, two packets of nuts and a bag of chocolate buttons (where did she think we were, a cinema?).

The clock on the wall ticked round to 10a.m. and we turned our papers over. I was obviously in the wrong exam, sitting the wrong paper and toyed with the idea of pretending to faint. But as if by magic, the words rearranged themselves and they actually started to make sense.

Three hours later, and with a lot of padding and random waffling, I was done. I clicked my pen off and shuffled the papers together. As I left, I noticed the woman sadly pack her teddy away. I stumbled out the building, high on relief and headed home to google Esping Anderson.

18th October 2013

In The Company Of Giants

The MS Society Awards 2013 at The Dorchester yesterday were, in the words of The Teenager, just awesome. To be in the same room as so many incredible people with so many inspiring stories and achievements is impossible to convey and to be a finalist in the same category as St Bartholomew's Hospital and Shift.ms was humbling.

I had no expectation of winning and was over the moon to receive a 'highly commended' certificate and bottle of bubbly. There's far too many highlights to mention, so here's a flavour of how the day unfolded:

We arrived early enough for The Teenager to be photographed posing next to a £1 million Bugati parked outside the hotel which he quickly tweeted to his friends. A champagne reception was then the perfect way to meet new people and put faces to names before being ushered into the ballroom for lunch.

I was thrilled to be sitting next to Joseph Carter, the acting Director of MS Society Cymru and on the same table as David Baker from St Bartholomew's Hospital with whom I had a lively and illuminating discussion about Alemtuzumab.

Lunch was superlative, the surroundings beautiful, but most importantly, the awards were emotional, moving and thoroughly well-deserved. The final announcement, for the MS Lifetime Achievement Award went to our very own Stuart Nixon (hardly a dry eye in the room).

The Teenager was busy having his photograph taken with as many celebrities as he could find - a big thank you to Stephanie Millward for signing autographs for him and letting him hold an Olympic torch. In all the excitement, I forgot to take any photographs myself (d'oh!), but the day passed in a whirlwind.

It was brilliant to have people come up to me, have a quick glance at my shoes and ask if I was Stumbling In Flats. To be told how much people loved my blog was an award in itself and I'm still floating on a high (possibly also due to the champagne...). What can I say? I truly was in the company of giants.

If the future of MS is in their hands - through research, through fundraising, through volunteering - then we are in very safe hands indeed.

20th October 2013

What Was I Saying Again?

'It's there, that watchermacallit on the thingiemabob. Next to the dooby-doo.' This was me yesterday, explaining to The Teenager where an important form he needed for school was.

MS has been having lots of fun with my brain and it's only getting worse (it's got absolutely nothing to do with turning 40 of course). I just can't seem to remember the most simple of words. I'll pause mid-sentence, sifting through years of education in my mind before finally landing on the word I'm looking for, so happy to have found it that I'll inappropriately yell out 'banana! I meant, banana!' Or some other word that completely escaped me five minutes earlier.

I also make up new words. Like last week when my mum asked me what I had planned that morning. 'Oh, it's flab day', I replied. She sighed and said, 'oh sweetheart, I know you're unhappy with your weight, but think positively. Have you tried chick peas?' I had to tell her that I was indeed unhappy with my weight, but I was actually going for my flu jab.

In my glory days, I prided myself on being able to converse in three languages (four if you count Glasgwegian). Now, I can barely get by with one.

Plus, I also have the ignominy of repeating myself, thanks to bizarre short term memory loss. I am in danger of turning into the dinner party guest from hell, the one that's invited along for a bit of comic relief.

I have visions of Christmas Day twenty years from now, with The Teenager taking his children to one side and gently reminding them to be patient with Granny Stumbling and not to laugh when she can't remember the punchlines to jokes, or when she asks them for the umpteenth time how they're doing in school. Just re-fill her sherry glass and hand her a copy of People's Friend. And under no circumstances are you to bring out Pictionary or Scrabble.

For now, although socially dire, I manage as best I can. In shops, when I can't remember what I went in for, I'll look at my watch and dash off, pretending I'm late for some appointment. In restaurants, I'll point to the menu, as if my mind is on higher things than ordering lunch. And when I'm out with friends, I'll....hang on, what was I saying again?

24th October 2013

Paper Round (And Round)

In my day (here we go again), I had a job when I was
14. So when The Teenager turned the same age in August,
we had a little chat. I explained that had he been born 100
years ago, he'd be going down the coal mines as we live in
Wales. Luckily for him, that was no longer a viable option,
so he'd have to look for something else.

Last summer he set himself up as a car-washer, lugging
round a bucket and sponge, knocking on doors. He did
quite well until he got bored with windscreens and wheel
trims. So with my rousing speech ringing in his ears (it will
give you discipline! it's character-building! you'll be earning
your own money!), he went to the local newsagents and
signed himself up for a paper round. He also seems to
have signed me up too.

He started on Monday, along with probably the most
apocalyptic rain to hit in months. I waved him off at 6.30
a.m. (You can do it!), set my mobile ring tone to loud,
made a cup of coffee and waited. Sure enough, within nine
minutes, there was an anguished phone-call. 'Come and
rescue me, pleeeeeaaaaase. I'm soaking, I can't see anything
for the rain, my papers are wet and I wanna come home.'

I trudged out to the car and searched for him. There he
was, a miserable, hunched figure holding a luminous bag
bulging with undelivered papers. He'd managed to cram

283

three soggy newspapers through letterboxes then got lost in the maze of back streets.

I set the sat nav and we searched through the driving rain for the remaining houses. By the time we got back home, we were both thoroughly fed up. After we'd dried off, it was time for another chat (lecture). 'You should have done a recce the day before. You should have planned your route. Responsibility, discipline, blah, blah, blah.'

We finally came to a tearful agreement. Each day, he would find the next street on his route and I would meet him there, so by the end of the week, he could confidently do the round himself. I have my reservations how long he'll last. Just this morning I asked him what he would do when he was in London with his dad one weekend a month. Quick as you like, he replied, 'well, you'll do it for me, won't you?'

26th October 2013

I'm Not Failing, I'm Sleeping

I had one of those earth-shattering, life-changing moments of clarity the other day. I closed my eyes at 10am, just to have a quick cat nap. Two hours later, I woke up. I was incensed, maddened by the sheer waste of time and looked with dismay at my unaccomplished 'To Do' list.

As I stumbled into the kitchen to make a cup of strong coffee, tripping over the cat (she's tiny but deadly), I stopped in my tracks. MS fatigue. I expect everyone else to take me seriously about how debilitating it can be, how much of a real symptom it is. And yet... *I* don't.

Instead, I see it as a major inconvenience, something to be tolerated if I am to get through the day intact. It's a distraction, holding me back from my real life. Or is it? I take my other MS symptoms seriously and factor them in, so why don't I do the same with my most significant symptom, fatigue?

Over the last two years, I have railed against the pointlessness of all this sleep. I flounce to my sofa in anger, utterly fed up at yet another hour passing me by with absolutely nothing achieved. This had to change. Rather than getting angry, I am now going to start respecting this fatigue, just as I accept that nerve pain, foot drop and stumbling are part of my life now. I can't change it, so I will accord it the same respect.

The fatigue is my body's way of telling me to slow down, my brain needs a rest. I will view it as a valid symptom, not a major annoyance. I tried out this new way of thinking yesterday. I had some things to do in the morning, and could feel the fatigue creeping up.

Back home, my brain shut down. The To Do list was put to one side, I got my duvet out and fell asleep. I woke up feeling better, accepting that this is my life now. I can't change it, but I can change how I approach it. I can absorb it into my life or I can go on forever feeling angry and a failure. And you know what? I feel that in some way I have made peace with myself. I'm not failing any more.

7th November 2013

The Red-Eyed Monster

If jealousy has green eyes, guilt most definitely has red, judging by the number of tears I cried on Tuesday night.

The day started innocuously enough. I schlepped to work, planned dinner for later, joked around with the boss. Then blam, thwack. Whole-body weakness, a brain stuffed with cotton wool and a need to get home pronto. The boss let me go early and back home blind panic set in.

I couldn't cook dinner. I could barely stand and when I did, I was bouncing off the walls, so I called my mum for help. She rushed down, but The Teenager was adamant that he didn't want to sleep overnight at her house (no Sky Sports News). She stayed for a while instead, giving the cat some chewy treats, cheering us up, admiring The Teenager's new Nirvana poster and giving me a bit of space to panic some more.

All I wanted to do was go to bed, and not just for a nap. During the day, I sleep when I have to and The Teenager is either out or at school, but the evenings are different. And therein lies the problem and source of my overwhelming guilt.

I'm a single parent (violins at the ready) and The Teenager is an only child. It just wouldn't be fair to abandon him at 6 or 7pm. I know he's 14, but I grew up with ill parents (my dad and my stepfather) and am keenly aware of the fears this gave me as a child.

So what did I do? MS left me no choice. I crawled into bed at 7pm, crying my eyes out, leaving The Teenager downstairs with his homework and remote control. Ten hours later I woke up, guilt flooding back. Until I looked at all the tweets I'd been sent while I'd been sleeping. Lovely, supportive tweets from all around the world. I wasn't going through this alone.

So, I stumbled out of bed, woke The Teenager for his paper round and we had a little chat as he struggled to get his waterproof trousers on. After patting me on the head and telling me he was fine, he launched into a goal-by-goal account of a football match he'd watched with the cat. Then he bashfully admitted he'd read my Twitter feed last night and felt comforted by all the messages of support, and he too felt less alone. Just before he left for school, he said I was more than welcome to go to sleep early again, he'd just chat to my Twitter friends. Um....

9th November 2013

We're Bang On Trend

I'm chuffed to share with you that something most of us with MS have been doing, like forever, has now been designated a zetigeisty trend - 'socialising lite'.

Driven by impossibly busy New Yorkers/Londoners, this involves combining two or three activities to fit more into your life. Or in our case, to ensure that we can still keep up with our friends/hobbies/interests despite fatigue and other pesky physical symptoms getting in our way.

The secret of socialising lite is to make your free time work for you. For people with MS, this translates as making those rare pockets of energy work harder for us. Even before I knew this was an actual trend (ooh, get me, chuck me a copy of Elle), I'd already started to do this - like combining catching up with a good friend and a shopping trip to town or asking my mum to help me in the garden, having a natter and putting the world to rights over a glass of wine afterwards. Killing two birds with one stone, but in a good way.

I miss doing what I used to do spontaneously, so this is a great compromise. Plus there's an added bonus of still feeling that I'm part of life, of society. Spending so much time at home has made me more aware that I need to get out, even just for a short while.

A more extreme form of socialising-lite is time-capping friends, which at first glance might seem rude, but with all of us juggling busier lives it's much more acceptable. Long gone are the days I'd go out for whole evenings, so rather than become a hermit (tempting), I say to my friends that I'd really love to see them, so how about we try that new wine bar/café/restaurant/exhibition and catch up for an hour? I get to see a good friend and try a new experience.

Time-capping doesn't mean I don't enjoy spending time with my friends, it just means that I don't want to wait for both of us to be free for a couple of hours/when I've got energy/when I'm not pinned to the sofa with fatigue. My next plan is to combine exercise and friends. So if anyone would like to pop over and join me in staring at my kettlebell (aka the doorstop), willing it to move by telekinesis, you're more than welcome. You bring the biscuits, I'll put the kettle on...

19th November 2013

A Sense of Disconnection

Oh my days. Who knew that being with a much-reduced internet connection over the last week could be quite so traumatic? The Teenager has gone through a whole range of emotions, from full-blown panic ('how will I survive? I am utterly, totally disconnected') to deep depression ('wake me up when it's over').

I helpfully suggested he read a book or, I don't know, make something. I was smartly told that whilst that may be acceptable for old people like me who went through their teenage years *gasp* without the internet, he'd rather sit in McDonalds like a saddo all day where they at least have free wifi, thank you very much.

Anyway, we're back on track and a sense of normality has returned to our little cottage (it won't last). In other news over this quiet week:

> • I had a letter inviting me to my graduation ceremony next May and did I want to hire a cap and gown? Which means my degree results must be on their way, eek.

> • The Teenager gave up his paper round. Enough said. You really don't want to hear about it. Or the specially-extended lecture I gave him.

• My smartphone (so badly-named) decided to get in on the internet act and freeze at inopportune moments, leading to a telling-off at work. Boss - 'oi, get off your phone'. Me -' I'm not on it, I'm waiting for it to unfreeze'. Boss - 'right, no more coffee or chocolate at break times'. Me 'be right with you, boss.' To show how sorry I was, when the phone worked I sent him pictures of cats doing funny things as that always cheers him up.

• All the crafty bits I ordered for Christmas have arrived - candle wicks, wax pellets, craft knife, cutting mat, white card, Christmas essential oil, modelling clay and star-shaped cookie cutters. Much hilarity will ensue.

• The cat kindly left a birds head outside my back door. Which I stepped on.

While we have been surviving without much internet, my mum (62 years old and a great-grandmother) whizzed ahead of us. In between Skyping her sister in Scotland, she upgraded her phone from a brick-like Nokia to a Samsung all-singing, all-dancing model. The Teenager is quietly impressed, if a little jealous.

21st November 2013

Walking That Lonely Mile

A couple of months after MS first appeared, I had a conversation with my partner, telling him I knew the months/years ahead would be hard and I would understand if he wanted to leave. He did. Perhaps I shouldn't have been surprised.

A study from 2009 indicated that women with cancer or MS were more than six times as likely to become separated or divorced within an average of six months of being diagnosed as were men with similar health issues.

In fairness, our relationship at that time wasn't as strong as it once was and this could have been the proverbial straw. Following his abrupt departure, I slumped on the sofa, too stunned to cry. My entire life was falling apart and just making an effort to get through each day was made more difficult by MS dragging me backwards, numbing my limbs, forcing me to sleep and making every step fraught with anxiety.

I wasn't walking a lonely mile (or several), I was stumbling blindly along a malignant deviation of the path I thought I had once been on. Looking at it positively with hindsight though, by becoming suddenly single I now 'only' had to worry about myself and The Teenager and how we would deal with MS. In all honesty, it was perhaps easier than patching up a rocky relationship that seemed to be springing lesions as quickly as my brain scans did.

Looking at it in the depths of despair, it was truly, gobsmackingly wretched. My self-worth was rapidly plummeting, I spent night after night inwardly howling at the unfairness of it all. Who would want me now? I mean, really? Divorced single mother, wrong side of 35, oh and by the way, I have MS. Form an orderly queue and sign up here if you're interested.

Two years down the line, thanks to a Campath-induced remission, I am slowly getting back on track. It's been a horrendously lonely time and I probably wouldn't have started this blog had I had a partner at my side. It would have been lovely to have someone to offload to, to share the journey (awful word) with.

On a practical level, it would have been brilliant to have another adult in the house when times were bad and I battled to maintain our normal routine. I'm learning to live alone. It's not easy. At times it's achingly awful. But I know that when the right person comes along, I will be in a much stronger frame of mind. Form that queue, and don't mind me while I cross my fingers.

25th November 2013

Numb And Number

We certainly know how to enjoy ourselves in our little household. Yesterday, after some lovely chicken pie, my big toe went completely numb (I'm not saying the two are connected, but we're having lamb next Sunday).

Unable to keep this to myself, I nimbly/numbly stumbled into the living room and told The Teenager. 'I can't feel my big toe!! See (flick) nothing! Go on, you try.'

'Mum. You're weird. If you weren't my mum, you'd be the kind of person you tell me not to talk to.'

'Look, try this (finds a drawing pin), you be the neurologist. Just press it on to my toe.'

'*sigh* Did you feel that?'

'No! Weird, huh?'

'Feel that?'

'That was my ankle. It's fine. Give me that.'

I'm no stranger to numbness. One of my first symptoms was completely numb feet, making walking a painful and tedious exercise in tentative negotiation, often resulting in 'hilarious' trips, foot drop making matters even worse. I was on first-name terms with every pavement in the vicinity.

Since my last relapse, things have calmed down a bit, although my feet still constantly tingle and buzz. In fact, I can't remember the last time they didn't. If I could go back to that very last day of 'normal' feet, I'd wear 8 inch Jimmy Choos for 24 hours and dance 'til dawn. Then I'd box-frame them (using my glue gun, natch) and hang them on the wall.

Numbness is an odd sensation, and to other people it doesn't even sound like a troubling symptom, but it sure makes life.....interesting. If I hold a book for too long, numb fingers. Waking up in the morning, numb arms. Sit for too long, numb legs. No wonder The Teenager calls me Numb Numb.

But as with most of MS's weird and wonderful box of tricks, it's surprising how much I'm used to it now, especially dropping things. I am a past master. Like the other day when I was in a smart café having breakfast. You know, those places that don't just put your beans on the plate, they serve them in dinky little chrome buckets (why?). You can see where I'm going with this.

The thing flew out my hands, I caught it, smiled with relief, then it jumped back out my very loose grip and clattered across the floor. Raised eyebrows from the next table. The waitress rushed over, 'Is everything ok?' It was so tempting to say, 'pull up a chair love, this may take some time....'

28th November 2013

I Did It. *faints*

I check my emails most mornings while I wait for the kettle to boil. Nestled among the offers to give me £100,000 if only I hand over my bank details to a very polite and sincere gentleman in Nigeria, lay the email I had been waiting for. 'Degree classification notice - please accept and confirm'.

My finger hovered over the email. The moment of truth, the culmination of six years study. I took a deep breath and clicked. Then I laughed. And hiccupped. Rushing to the printer to see actual proof before the email magically disappeared, I did a high five (ok, a very low two, but you know what I mean).

I am now the proud owner of a Bachelor of Science degree (with Honours, yay). An upper Second Class. A 2:1. Still can't believe it.

Thinking about it, I have studied for the last 10 years out of 11, my first qualification being a degree equivalent in Homeopathy (long story). My Glaswegian auntie, on seeing the letters I was eligible to use for that course (RSHom), said, 'oh dear, if you say that out loud with a Scottish accent, it sounds a wee bit rude, doesn't it?).

Well, now I'm a Bachelor(ette), which is rather fitting, given my present singledom. I'm supposed to attend a graduation ceremony next May, donning a cap and gown and walking up to a stage to accept a bit of paper tied nicely with a ribbon. I'll sign up, but the logistics of doing this in front of hundreds of people will be left for another time.

It sounds weird, but this achievement is the positive culmination of a terrible couple of years. The last two years of the degree were excruciating. My brain died a slow death, slinking out of the room without a backwards glance or apology. I struggled with every single aspect of the course. I came so, so close to giving it all up.

What was once fairly easy for me (I'm an unabashed girly swot), became unintelligible nonsense. Essays were torture. In tutorials, I sat with a slightly astonished look on my face.

But I didn't give up and I'm proud of myself. I didn't give up during the diagnostic process, during the legal proceedings against my ex-employer who sacked me for the heinous crime of having MS, during two lots of Campath treatment and their after effects. I did it. I actually did it.

2nd December 2013

Life Sure Ain't Like The Movies

A funny thing happened the other day. I was lying on
the sofa reading a book, plucking Maltesers from a box I'd
craftily hidden from The Teenager. The next thing I knew
I had woken with a start, the book (and Maltesers) having
crashed to the floor.

This may sound boringly insignificant, but I thought
stuff like that only happened in movies for dramatic effect
- just like you can see the Eiffel Tower from any window
in Paris. I ranted to the cat after she'd stopped chasing the
Maltesers round the floor - how could anyone fall asleep
so quickly that they couldn't put their book down first?

Either explanation is most unpalatable: a) old age
creeping up on me b) worsening MS fatigue. Mind you, if
my life were a movie, there would be a conveniently-placed
handsome man who would gently prise the book from my
fingers, wrap me in a cashmere blanket and gaze upon my
slumbering face before dimming the lights and nestling
another log on the open fire.

Furthermore, kindly neighbours would have left a pile
of casseroles and lasagnas outside my door during my
worst relapses two years ago. They would also have
surprised me by putting up my Christmas tree and
arranging for an angelic choir to sing carols outside my
door, snow falling softly.

On recovery, I would magically spring the money to spend a month somewhere exotic to 'find myself'. There would be shots of me wandering sadly down golden-sand beaches. Towards the end however, I would be laughing and learning important, life-affirming lessons from the wise natives, arriving back home with a new-found sense of purpose in life. But life isn't like the movies.

When I woke and found my book and chocolates on the floor, I was cold, I hadn't started dinner and I found The Teenager hanging off an open fridge door bemoaning the lack of junk food ('everyone else in school gets to have it, why not me, you meanie? What am I supposed to do with a tangerine?').

I explained to him what had happened. He was unperturbed ('Mum, you're, like, old, you know? It's what old people do, my grandad does it all the time').

Out of interest, I asked him what he would like to see come true from the movies. He didn't hesitate - 'one of those huuuuuuuge American fridges crammed with junk food and my own den in the basement and … (I stopped listening after five minutes)......

5th December 2013

And Here's One I Made Earlier

Who knew crafternoons could be so stressful? I had a couple of days off work recently, and inspired by countless articles in picture-perfect Christmas magazines, I had amassed a whole pile of crafty bits just perfect for creating a home-made Christmas.

Getting into an arty festive mood, I put some Christmas carols on, brewed some cranberry herbal tea, tied my hair up in a scarf, and set to. After an exhausting afternoon spent weeping into my glitter, here's what I learned:

- Invisible thread is called invisible thread for a reason.

- Air-drying clay does not dry in 24 hours.

- The cat likes licking air-drying clay (eeeew).

- Metal star-shaped cookie cutters are painful.

- Potato stamping isn't half as much fun at 40 as it was at 4.

- Paper folding is not relaxing.

- Cutting card with a craft knife is deadly.

- Too much herbal tea was a mistake.

- The magazines lied.

I don't give up that easily, so the next afternoon, I put some hard rock music on, made some mulled wine and wrapped my hair tightly with an elastic band (glue guns and hair don't mix).

First up, the easy one. Slice some oranges, put in oven at a low heat for four hours ('a delightful aroma will infuse your home with a wondrous Christmas spirit'). Next, glue-gun some baubles to a distressed wooden frame, in the shape of a Christmas tree (a simple, yet charming idea). Finally, make your own candles ('a bee-yoootiful gift for friends and family').

My oranges curled up and died, sending out plumes of evil-smelling, acrid smoke, I became more distressed than my baubles and frame and after boiling up wax pellets for the candles, I realised too late that the wicks I had ordered were too short.

All I have to show for my efforts is a string of clay stars. After all the pummelling, rolling out, cutting out, three days of air-drying and chasing the cat away from them, I was determined not to be beaten.

The next day, I went to Poundland (three fold-out stars for a quid), chucked out all my magazine articles, cursed Kirstie Allsopp and Pinterest and flopped on the sofa to watch 'Elf' for the eighth time (with some re-heated mulled wine).

17th December 2013

Um, Om?

After a week which saw my stress levels catapulted into the stratosphere, I thought it was time to chill out, breathe deeply and relax. A spot of meditation perhaps?

Call me a sceptic, but both my 'journeys' into meditation have been unmitigated disasters. The first time, I signed up for a class to impress a new partner. Big mistake. The session was led by a wild-haired woman dressed in a flowing dress and beads, perched on a dais high above, beaming down upon us lesser mortals. A self-styled guru who had changed her name from Brenda to something vaguely spiritual-sounding.

She promised to share with us the mystical training she had received over the last hundred years and travels through several continents (by donkey). I left after three hours and split up with the partner not long after.

A few years later, I tried again, this time when I was living in Norway. At the introduction session I was told I would be given my very own meditation 'word' by another guru, a ruddy, wild-haired man dressed in a flowing silk shirt and beads. The word would be whispered to me and I would use it as a focus to help clear my mind.

Unfortunately, the word imparted to me in Norwegian sounded very rude in English and I burst out laughing which was not particularly enlightened of me.

Would I be third time lucky? I already take time out each morning to mentally floss my brain, so how would I fare sitting still with a blank mind? Thanks to MS, that's actually not particularly hard. My brain is frequently blank, tumbleweed blowing past and I sit down an awful lot anyway.

I read up on it, took ten minutes out and sat in a quiet place. My neighbour started drilling next door, the cat yelled for more food and I heard my post being delivered. But that was ok, I was supposed to listen to the noise, my mind would get bored and would naturally move on.

Then it was all about counting my breathing, so if my mind wandered, I could pull it back in and focus again. After ten minutes, I opened my eyes, glared at the cat and asked myself how I felt. To be honest, not that bad at all. Will I continue the good work? Probably not.

19th December 2012

MS Christmas Survival Guide

Christmas is the one time in the year us peeps with MS can really blend in. Over the next two weeks, it will be perfectly socially acceptable for me to nod off at odd times of the day, stumble and talk gibberish.

Last Christmas, I fell up the stairs, followed by a round of applause. However, a little forward- planning is still essential, so here is my quick guide to surviving the festive frolics:

> • Internet shopping - it's still not too late! I have not had to brave any crowds, queue for hours or fight over the last Christmas pudding. Plus, I have a rather handsome postman I have seen so often I'm sure the neighbours think I'm having a clandestine affair (I wish).

> • Sleep - make the most of this time. No need to explain why you've dozed off in front of the telly for the third time that day, or fallen asleep face-down in your turkey dinner. People will laugh rather than gasp. They may even take a photo and put it on Twitter. Instant fame guaranteed.

> • Stumbling/tripping - let's face it, everyone will be doing a lot of this. It's practically mandatory. Why not have a festive quiz? If you trip, turn to your assembled family and say, 'aha! Now was that MS or

the extra-strong mulled wine?' Winner gets the last purple Quality Street.

• Cog fog - this is especially handy during Christmas. When (not if) a family argument starts and you're asked if Auntie Doreen really did say that terrible thing about Auntie Doris thirty years ago, just put on your most tragic expression and tell Auntie Dot that you're a hopeless case, you can't even remember what you had for dinner yesterday.

• Extra help - if you're having a bad MS day, waylay a passing small(ish) child and tell them you want to play a game. Little kids love dressing up and pretending, so why not pop an apron on them and tell them you'll give them two quid if they play at being a maid, like in Downton Abbey. That way you can have a steady stream of Twiglets, refills, magazines and chocolates delivered straight to your sofa. Plus you get extra Brownie points for entertaining a child for seven hours.

So, I wish you all a very merry (hic) Christmas. Hold your heads up high (with a sneaky peek at your feet), go forth and celebrate.

27th December 2013

MS Doesn't Take A Holiday

Well, the big day has come and gone. Shame I can't say the same about MS, which had the bad grace to leave a few extra presents under the tree.

It started so well. We had our company Christmas bash - just me and the boss marooned in a restaurant full of proper office parties (all excruciatingly forced jollity, loud voices and a solitary woman crying in the loos).

We had a glass of wine at my place afterwards, where I amused the boss by holding up the plastic wineglasses my mum bought me for Hallowe'en after I smashed my last one. 'Spooky ghost or howling skull?'. Awkward.

The next day I had champagne with the family while The Teenager was in London. I took it easy, inwardly congratulating myself but MS had other ideas. The last thing I remember is getting home, feeding the cat, tripping over, hitting my head on the door and knocking myself out.

I woke up several hours later with the cat next to me shaking her head sadly. Then my arms started to go numb at inopportune moments. Normally it's one or the other, along with constantly buzzing legs and feet. So with two numb arms and dodgy legs, Christmas Day was a trial.

We helped to serve Christmas lunch to a roomful of pensioners. Someone thrust a jug of gravy into my hands and motioned for me to go forth and pour. Gripping the jug as tightly as I could, I made my way round. I did try to explain that gravy washes out of clothes quite easily, just pop a bit of Vanish on first, but they were unimpressed and a good few elderly ladies glared at me as they dabbed ineffectually at their skirts and blouses.

So now we are in that odd period between Christmas and New Year. Numb arms or not, I have still managed to polish off a tub of Quality Street (the pain was worth it). I fall asleep at odd times of the day, I've tripped over a stray bauble and am considering installing grab rails in the shower (you really, really don't want to hear that story).

MS has certainly made Christmas that little bit more interesting. Laugh? 'Til I cried.

29th December 2013

You Can't Argue With MS

Along with sprouts, bad telly and a chocolate overdose, Christmas just wouldn't be Christmas without a few arguments. I now know I will never win another one as long as MS insists on using my brain as Play Doh.

I used to be quite good at thinking on my feet, remembering the punchlines to jokes and telling anecdotes without losing the thread halfway through. I could also hold my own pretty well in an argument or disagreement. Those days have passed and I now sit with a slightly perplexed look on my face as I work out my response to a point made ten minutes earlier. In the spirit of fairness, I reckon us peeps with MS should be given a few allowances when it comes to arguing:

> • We should be given prior notice, giving us time to think of some clever and witty retorts.
>
> • We should be allowed to take notes during the aforementioned argument. A personal scribe should be allotted if, like me, your handwriting is now worse than your neurologist's.
>
> • We should be granted 'argument breaks', allowing us time to gather our thoughts (and energy). Lucozade should be supplied as standard.

• Similarly, a sofa should be made available if we start yawning, and the argument rescheduled for a more convenient time.

I'm resigning myself to the fact that I am now a pushover when it comes to arguing, although when The Teenager starts one (all too frequently over this festive season), I end up falling back on that age-old parent phrase - 'because I said so'. Which isn't very original, but you can't argue with that one. This is normally followed by The Teenager storming upstairs and blasting out his music.

To be honest, I don't really miss point-scoring and the hollow victory of winning every argument. My initial frustration has given way to calm acceptance and I have now added it to my list of things I have lost, along with heels and staying up past my bedtime. So the next time an argument brews, I will stumble inelegantly away or just stay put and use one of The Teenager's favourite phrases, 'talk to the hand'..

3rd January 2014

I Resolve To Be Totes Amazeballs

A very Happy New Year to everyone! At the stroke of midnight on the 31st, I threw off the debris of a long year and became instantly regenerated. A bit like Doctor Who. It's exhilarating to wipe the slate clean and imagine how much better this year will be.

This euphoria generally lasts until the 3rd or 4th of January when we realise we're still the same old person. Sigh. Anyway, this year I resolve to be totes amazeballs, at least until the end of the month. My resolutions are:

- Stop using youth slang. Oops.

- Embrace every challenge rather than hiding under my duvet.

- Master the art of cooking rice (yup, this was on my list last year too).

- Learn to play the saxophone.

- Work out what I want to be when I grow up.

I got the chance to try out two of these when my oven died a slow death. With an Ocado delivery packed with oven-cook food on its way and The Teenager due back on

Saturday, it was a mini crisis. But I remained calm and avoided the duvet temptation.

To cut a very long story short (tears and foot stamping), it will be fixed today and I can now cook rice as the hob works fine. Life is slowly getting back to normal after the bright lights of Christmas. School starts back on Monday, the washing machine will once more be pushed into full service and I will bear witness to every high and low of The Teenager's football team. I know far more about the Premier League than I ought to.

So here's to 2014 and all that it will fling at us. This will be the first year in a long while I am not a) waiting for an MS diagnosis b) being bullied at work c) being sacked for having MS d) coming to terms with an MS diagnosis. Totes fab.

10th January 2014

Plots And Plans

When I was first diagnosed with MS, a trusted health professional asked me, 'so when will you be giving up work then?' An outdated concept perhaps, but it got worse. By the end of the fateful day I disclosed my MS at work, plans were underway to get rid of me as quickly as possible. Just over a year later, and after not taking the very obvious hints, I was unceremoniously sacked on a dreary Monday morning.

Work and MS. It hasn't really been a great story for me so far. On the bright side though, my friend has been employing me for over a year now while I still look for a new job.

The downside is he doesn't run a cool café or bijoux boutique, but a construction company. I normally work from home doing boring thrilling admin (pyjamas, toast and cat - hope the boss isn't reading), but sometimes, if I promise to behave, he allows me on site.

This week, I was allowed out to drive a mini dumper truck. Basically sitting down all day, tootling up a lane and back. Not that different from sitting down all day tootling to the kitchen and back, except I had an emergency stop button and the coffee was lousy.

I was given a quick lesson first, 'this is stop, this is go and this is a steering wheel.' Yup, got it. Woolly hat on and

I was ready to go. To cut a long story short, it's not that exciting after the first couple of goes. The highlight of my day was waving to a toddler who was peering through the window shouting 'Bob! It's Bob the Builder! But mummy, it's a girl!'

Anyway, as I was tootling along, I realised I really should get a proper job. I've tried, I really have. I'm signed up to all the job sites, I scroll through pages and pages of thrilling career opportunities but still there is nothing out there. I've moved seamlessly from being restricted by childcare commitments to being restricted by MS.

I know I'm lucky. I couldn't ask for a better boss, I've learned a huge amount and can now read architectural plans like a pro. But plans are afoot. I can't go far in the construction world when I can't even go up a ladder.

But you know what? I'll miss the bacon sarnies, the camaraderie and the filthy jokes. What other job can offer all that?

13th January 2014

Ikea. That Is All

The Teenager needed a desk, so we bit the bullet and
drove to the big blue box on Sunday.

'Mum, why is Ikea, like, all yellow and blue?'

(weeps into steering wheel) 'Er, Swedish flag?'

We parked up alongside thousands of others and joined
the masses who were swarming through the doors. Only
the café was open so we followed the same masses to the
restaurant. One rubbery-looking bargain breakfast (The
Teenager) and a grotty coffee (me) later, we got in line to
follow the infuriating, snaking queue past everything we
didn't want until we got to the desks.

Ikea appears to be a destination of choice for
wandering tribes of families clutching bags of tea lights
and pushing empty ankle-snapping trollies, smugly
superior in the knowledge that they watch Scandi-dramas
on BBC4 every weekend with a few bottles of Swedish
beer. 'Oh, decisions, decisions! Should we go for the (very
bad Swedish accent) Glivarp or the Norden table? But, oh,
the Melltorp is divine....darling, did you pick up the tea
lights?'

Anyway, desk. Sorted. Scribble down where to pick it
up. Swivel chair? Check. Onto the pleasantly-named
Market Hall where I whisked The Teenager swiftly
through to the bay where he attempted to lift a couple of

one-tonne boxes onto a wonky trolley. Joined the long queue, where The Teenager decided to abandon me and buy an ice cream ('had to, only 25p').

Pay, pick up a couple of catalogues (hard currency among my friends) and join the masses at the supersized lifts. Car, struggle, swearing. Home. Then comes the fun bit. Let's just say, who knew a swivel chair could be broken down in to 150 different components? Who knew I would break down, allen key in sweaty hand, wishing I had bought another packet of mini Daim bars to soften the blow?

Chucked the cat out of the discarded boxes. Cried a little bit more. Chucked the allen key against the wall. Finally, desk assembled (drawer's a tad loose but don't tell The Teenager, it's dark in his bedroom, he won't notice).

End result - one Happy Teenager (shock). One shell-shocked parent. I was reminded of a van I saw on the motorway last year. Their slogan was 'Why DIY?' Why indeed....

21st January 2014

Disarmed

I think I got a bit carried away with the dumper truck in work last week. The steering wheel has a funny knobbly thing on it, so I happily swung it round and round, little realising the damage it would do to my arm and wrist.

Fast forward a couple of days and I'm in agony. I've sprained my right arm and I am once more off work. Getting to be a bit of a habit?

The Teenager has been pressed into service like never before - laundry, getting dishes out the oven, sweeping through the house. Much wailing and gnashing of teeth, 'I am *not* your servant' (stomp stomp) being a favourite retort, with me responding, 'Oi! I can still flick the internet off with one finger, so ner, ner, ner, ner, ner.'

Anyway, I am moping around the house feeling rather sorry for myself. Who knew arms could be so useful? There is so much I just can't do without reaching for the painkillers and 'ooofing' out loud. Shampooing my hair is farcical. Driving is off-limits and holding a book to read is deadly. I feel as if I've been snowed-in without the 'yay, we're in the middle of a national crisis!' excitement that follows half an inch of the white stuff.

I took the bus into town yesterday to meet friends for a sushi lunch, and try as I might, I just can't use chopsticks left-handed. So I gave it a go with my right, wincing, and I just about managed (I was hungry - 6 plates). I've bought myself a tubi-grip wotsit and it helps a little. I've weaned myself off the strong painkillers after I started dreaming whilst awake. In short, I am Fed Up.

The upside is, I have cleaned out the 'whatever' drawer, compiled an Amazon wish list, caught up with all the subtitled programmes on my Sky Planner and got to grips (ha!) with my 'iPad for Complete and Utter Idiots' book. I am now semi-fluent in Danish and Swedish and have found my can opener. Plus I have a bunch of useless apps.

I had to text in sick this morning, something I hate doing. The boss responded, 'no worries, we're having a lovely fry-up in the cafe'. Meh. If the promise of that won't get me back to work, nothing will.

25th January 2014

I've Gone Over To The Mac Side

The idea of using an iPhone used to fill me with horror. With my MS dodgy sausage fingers, the teeny-weeny keyboard would be next to useless, unless I wanted to send texts saying, 'hmjjf keleow gdder'.

I had a Blackberry, ideal as the buttons are raised. Doing my research when it was time to upgrade, I stumbled into a phone shop. The salesperson was most unhelpful. 'You want to stay with Blackberry? Hey guys, this lady wants a Blackberry!'

He explained in disparaging terms (not hiding his sniggers very well) that they didn't even sell them anymore, and would I want a phablet instead? Big buttons. Yeah, but a huge block of a thing I'd feel a right banana talking on.

Anyway, the boss solved the problem. He bought me an iPad mini for Christmas so I could be more productive in work ('we can sink our stuff!' Huh?). He gleefully told me I now had no option but to upgrade to an iPhone. Well, I was petrified. I took home the shiny new phone. The Teenager was impressed - '4G ready, like, mint.' He stroked the phone reverently. He laughed at my pink stylus and warned me to buy a case pronto - 'mum, dur, like you drop everything.' Fair point.

A week later, I am smitten. I don't do things by half, so I bought a book and slowly worked my way through it.

Maybe I shouldn't have face-timed the boss at 10pm last night though, just to test it out. I waved at him and admired his pyjamas.

I've downloaded a bunch of apps. I like most of them apart from the weight-loss one. I diligently add my weight every day and it informed me this morning that the date I would reach my desired weight would be 2023.

The keyboard is very patient with me, correcting all my typing mistakes and Siri answers all my questions. I told it the other day, 'I love you' and it replied 'that's nice. Can we get back to work now?' I then asked, 'what's better, a Blackberry or an iPhone?' The answer was, 'Oh Stumbling, I'm all Apple, all the time.'

28th January 2014

Don't Mention The 'V' Word

During the first week of January (when I went to stock up on Creme Eggs), I briefly thought about boycotting my local newsagent.

On leaving the store I was brutally confronted with a huge display under the banner 'Winter Essentials'. Alongside the de-icer, Arctic-proof gloves and those grip things you attach to your shoes, was a stand full of Valentine's cards, plastic red roses and cheap teddies holding sateen hearts. Pah. So having a significant other is now a Winter Essential? Double pah.

Not long after, I had an email offering me and my significant other a 'truly romantic experience on that most romantic day of the year' at my local gastro-pub. A glass of cheap sparkling wine on arrival, a wilted red rose for 'the lady' and a three course lovingly-prepared meal to 'tingle the palate'. And all for only £42 a head. Are they having a laugh?

The evil-singleton side of me toyed with the idea of schlepping along on that most romantic of days, sitting in the bar and watching awkward couples crammed into the restaurant. But that's a bit mean. Isn't it? Maybe I should launch myself back onto the dating scene? There's a few problems with that though:

• MS

• I still dress like a student and don't wear strappy heels. And I haven't mastered the art of a sophisticated up-do.

• I would yawn my way through dates, and not solely because my companion is regaling me with tales of his pot-holing.

• MS

• I still need to lose a few ~~pounds~~ stone.

• MS

My friends and family are very encouraging though. 'It's not about the MS, it's about you, who you are.' 'You have lovely eyes.' (what they say to fat people). And my ever-adoring son, 'Have you sent off your application for the next series of The Undateables yet?'

Well I reckon we should scrap Valentine's Day. Let's have a new celebration, Singleton Day. This would involve buying an M&S meal-deal for a tenner (including a bottle of wine) and scoffing/quaffing the whole lot on our own, with 'I Will Survive' playing on a loop in the background.

We could encourage our friends to send us boxes of chocolates to help us ease the pain. Three layers of mascara would be an essential, all the better to show our tears with. So spare a thought for us sad, lonely, slipper-wearing, talking-to-the-cat peeps. And all donations of recycled men gratefully received.

30th January 2014

Catching Me When I'm Falling

Hours, days, weeks can go by and I'm absolutely fine. I have a good life. MS is under control (just about) and no longer scares the living daylights out of me. I sometimes struggle to remember what life was like before it.

So why do I have moments when I plunge into a deep, black depression? Just like MS, there is no way of knowing when it will strike. I can have had the best of days, life is on track and the future is looking a shade more defined than before. Then suddenly the shutters come down, blocking out the light.

This sensation is like a relapse of the mind - a sudden, catastrophic descent into despair. I'm aware it's happening, just like physical relapses when there is a period of disconnection before the symptoms flare up, snatching control of my body away from me. I know people with MS are more likely to experience depression, whether due to our circumstances or from our brains playing havoc with our minds.

Whatever the explanation, I need to find ways to cope with this. Perhaps it's been around since MS started but I was unable to distinguish it from the shock of the diagnosis. Now life has reached a happier plateau, maybe I can see it in unsplendid isolation.

When it happens, I want to retreat, hide myself away and wait until it passes. But life gets in the way. I have a Teenager to raise and a house to run. I have a life. My friends and family are unfortunately becoming used to helping me pick up the pieces. They catch me and hold onto me so I don't fall any further.

They don't try to cheer me up or tell me how much worse it could have been. They are simply there for me. If I knew how to fix this, I would. It's an unwelcome visitor in the new life I'm constructing for me and my little family. It lifts as suddenly as it comes. Colours burst through once more and life is shiny, exciting and vibrant again. I am trying. I can't retreat, but I can sit out the storm.

7th February 2014

Dragging My Feet

You know when you wake up with a brand spanking-new MS symptom? That heart-stopping moment when all your worst fears come crashing in on you? Yup. This happened last week.

A normal morning - coffee, cat, catch-up with paperwork, countdown to waking The Teenager. Except that morning was different. My normally-good foot refused to play fair. It gave up the ghost, schlepping behind me like a stroppy Teenager (and boy, do I have experience of *that*). Panic rose and I quelled it.

The next day, same thing. And the next. A new symptom. Probably every person with MS's worst nightmare. I decided to beat it at its own game, determinedly lifting the naughty foot with every step. Only problem was, I looked ever so slightly odd. Exaggerated. Like I was walking in slow motion to the 'Chariots of Fire' theme tune.

I ran it past the MS nurse (the problem, not my foot) but declined an appointment. 'I'll be fine!' I ran it past the chiropractor who urged me to call the MS team. 'I'll be fine!' I put it out my mind.

But it stayed and I dragged my foot round the house. Finally, I took the offered appointment. What's worse? Being told it may be a relapse or it may not be a relapse? It doesn't really matter either way, I won't take any more steroids. I can't bear the thought of waking up at 2am and having a strong compulsion to dust all the lightbulbs and clean the skirting boards, such is the bizarre energy those tiny tablets give me. Plus they destroy taste buds. And I pack on the weight no matter how many edamame beans I eat.

So I am in a kind of weird limbo. I worry that the endless relapses have found a sneaky way through the Campath treatment I had. I worry about my mobility - the defining point of being accepted as 'relatively normal' within societal boundaries. Above all, my dodgy, annoying, schlepping foot has dominated the last week. I am panicking. Ever so slightly.

9th February 2014

Dodging The Bullet

Well it seems the draggy, schleppy foot is here to stay for a little while longer. It's surprising how quickly I've got used to it, the exaggerated lifting of the offending foot. Apart from The Teenager mimicking the Kennedy Space Center voice - 'One giant leap for woman....'

Anyway, I've been thinking. It could be an old symptom coming back in a sneaky, evolved form, or it could be a new symptom. I could tie myself up in knots about it. Like most of us with MS, I spend my days inwardly saying, 'there goes the foot drop, oh, that'll be the heat intolerance and yup, some loss of balance for good measure.' And, 'can I go to sleep now?'

Maybe I spend so much time in fear of a new symptom, a relapse, a further loss, that I forget to concentrate on the here and now. The MS symptoms will go their own way regardless. The way my mind goes is of my own choosing. Over that, at least, I have a modicum of control.

So maybe I should stop worrying about dodging the bullet. If it happens, it happens. I was utterly paralysed by fear last week. And what good did it do me? I came down with a stomach bug. In a way, it was a relief to concentrate on a non-MS symptom for once. All thoughts of MS were pushed out my mind as I put my much-diminished energy in to becoming better as quickly as possible.

I crawled back into bed, the monotony of it only relieved by my friend delivering me all the Saturday newspapers, a McDonald's burger and Coke (I know, I know, but it helped) and a big bar of chocolate.

If this last week has taught me anything at all, it is that MS is part of who I am. The more I try to side-swerve and ignore what is happening, the more I suffer when a symptom comes to the fore. It's not about giving in, but accepting that it happens. The meltdown I went through was probably far worse than the symptom itself. And what does that show me? It is my mind, not my body that is out of control. A sobering thought.

13th February 2014

Teenage Tantrums

Our little house is in a state of uproar. To begin with, I trusted The Teenager to go to the hairdresser on his own. He's fond of the woman who cuts his hair and he's partial to the lollipops (meant for the little kids, not six foot 14 year olds), so I thought I'd leave him to it.

Off he went. Within half an hour, a photo pinged to my phone. A selfie of The Teenager, pretty much bald. And I had paid a tenner for the privilege.

Then Parents' Evening. Or rather, lack of it. After last year's disaster (a complete and utter bun-fight), I asked him to kindly request that his teachers email me their reports. MS heat intolerance and unsteadiness on my feet make it nigh on impossible to queue-hop and use my elbows effectively. I waited. And waited.

Hey, you're teachers haven't emailed me yet.' 'Oh, computer servers must be down again (rolls eyes) you know what it's like.' 'Hmmm.' I waited some more. 'Oh, there's a terrible bug going round. Like, no one's in school. Hoooooonestly.' 'Hmm.' I called the school.

'Oh yes, you are the mother of The Teenager?' 'Um, yes.' 'Ahhhh.' Right. Yes. We have a few, well, issues.'

I explained what I thought I had organised. 'Hah! (foolish parent). Anyway, an email was sent out to all the teachers, asking them to get in touch with their thoughts about my son. Let's just say it wasn't pleasant.

When he got home from school that day, I brandished a wad of printed off emails at him and demanded answers.

'All the teachers hate me. S'not my fault.'

'Why has one teacher said 'he appreciates the difficulties with regards The Teenager attending after school training?' You live a couple of hundred metres from the school. What're you saying??'

(furtive, shifty look) 'Dunno.'

Anyway, to cut a fraught story short, I reminded him that I did not spend an entire Sunday putting together a flat-pack desk from Ikea, just for him to put his telly on it. And the lovely little lamp I got him. Or the executive chair.

'And why are you answering your teachers back?'

'Dunno. They said I wouldn't get any qualifications so I asked to see theirs.'

I was a girly swot in school. I have no idea where he gets this attitude from. What annoys me is that he can do it if he puts his mind to it. We had The Discussion. About how he was throwing away his future. 'I'm not! Alan Sugar started off selling stuff from the back of his car.'.

Give me strength.

17th February 2014

For The Last Time

Many moons ago. when I held my colicky, screaming baby in my arms, a visitor smiled indulgently at me, took another sip of their tea and said, 'Ahhh, make the most of it, they grow up so fast.' I glared at them through glazed and dull eyes. Oh really. Infinity stretched ahead of me, filled with nappies, screaming, cabbage leaves (don't ask) and snatched sleep.

Fourteen years down the line, I now know what they mean. The years whizzed by. I visited a five-day old baby last week and was just about to say, 'Ahh, make the most of it....' but I held my tongue. Instead, I stared in awe at the tiny bundle, stunned that The Teenager had once been that size.

I remember all the firsts. The first step (far, far too soon), the first word ('food'), the first day at nursery, at primary, at secondary. The first time he stayed over at a friend's house. The first time he made a Lego kit by himself.

The sadness is, I never knew when the endings would be. The last time he held my hand crossing the road, or the last time he wanted a colouring-in book. We don't know until time passes and we realise they took place some time ago.

Excuse me for being a touch maudlin. I guess I'm just a bit angry that a lot of 'last times' took place during the turmoil of the MS diagnosis. Whether I liked it or not, The Teenager had to come to terms with a parent who has a long-term illness, with his dad living 140 miles away.

Don't get me wrong, I never put an unacceptable responsibility on too-young shoulders. I strove to maintain our normal routine, even when it was beyond-exhausting. But inevitably life changed, and so suddenly.

Gone was the parent with boundless energy, who would go on long day trips, packing the car up and heading off. Gone was the spontaneity, the feeling that yeah, we can do that, why not? Instead, life was filled with, 'not now', 'maybe tomorrow'.

I've never lost sight of him though. He is central in everything I do, hence the Campath treatment. Who cares about the potential side effects when it can keep me on my feet?

Perhaps instead of thinking remorsefully about the 'last times', I should concentrate on the new experiences The Teenager has. The new 'firsts'. First razor, first girlfriend, first rain-sodden festival he goes to. Hang on, did I just say first girlfriend? Hmmm.

19th February 2014

A Double Diagnosis?

As if having the label of MS slapped on you isn't bad enough, there's another sneaky diagnosis that creeps up alongside it. That of the well-meaning hypochondriac.

I never really worried about my health in those halcyon pre-MS days. My body did what I told it to do, when I told it to. I had the usual sniffles and aches, just like anyone else. I even used to boast how strong my immune system must be as I rarely took a sick-day off work. How times have changed.

It probably all started after the first Official Relapse. I was urged to keep a symptom diary, noting down anything unusual or out of the ordinary. For the first time in my life, I was closely observing my body. Every single teeny-weeny symptom was duly logged and dated.

At the following appointment with the neurologist, he asked me about any recent symptoms. I took a deep breath and read through my list. Ten minutes later, with the neurologist no doubt planning his grocery list or clocking the cracks in the ceiling, I finished with 'oh, and my nose sometimes twitches AND my eyelid does too. Weird, huh?' In short, am I well on my way to becoming a full-blown hypochondriac?

Not that I pester the medical staff or take up endless appointments. I am reluctant to 'bother anyone'. I keep my anxiety to myself. But it's awfully tiring. Or is that the MS fatigue? It's very difficult to differentiate between MS and non-MS symptoms.

Some non-MS illnesses are made worse by MS, or at least, not helped. And am I more tired than usual because of work or because of MS? I could tie myself up in knots, if I had the energy. I think the problem is that a lot of us with MS live with the knowledge that we are only as good as our last relapse. We scan the horizon, waiting for the next bunch of symptoms to ride over the hill.

And speaking of over the hill, I probably need to remind myself that I have indeed reached the milestone age of 40. The age when bits don't work quite as well as they should. When we nod off in front of the telly. When we get creaky joints. Must dash (stumble). The tip of my finger has just gone numb, perhaps I'd better jot it down.....

8th March 2014

Dear MS

Dear MS,

Were you having a laugh? I used to speak three languages, yet that morning three years ago, I woke up unable to speak English. You threw sand in my eyes and made me walk funny. And I certainly didn't want to have that MRI, nor the medieval lumbar puncture that followed.

But, you know what? You're here now, so I might as well get used to having you around, you pesky minx, you. So, keep on making my hand numb (haha), keep on forcing me to sit down and fall asleep no matter what the situation (gah), keep on making me avoid any direct sunlight as if I were a vampire. You are a parasite and I hate you. You have ruined my life. But sadly, you are part of me now so we might as well get on.

I will accept the enforced sleep breaks, the dodgy walking, the tripping. But I will never, ever accept the worst you can throw at me. Who cares if I no longer speak fluent Norwegian? I can still read it, so ner ner ner ner ner. Who cares if I can no longer write 3000 word essays? I graduated last year. Yah. Boo.Sucks. You are a leech. You destroy everything you touch. Families, relationships, careers. You took everything from me and you were unrelenting in your destructive mission.

So you chewed me up and spat me out. I lost my partner, my job, my career, most of my friends. But I win. I will be a better Me. I didn't ask for you to appear and gnaw at my nerve endings. It's ironic. I feel you. I feel emotions. And that will not end, no matter what you throw at me.

Yours,

Stumbling

10th March 2014

MS Replies

Dear Stumbling,

Thank you for your kind and thought-provoking letter (see, I do read your blog, so ner ner ner ner ner, as you so eloquently put it).

I think it's time we had a little chat, don't you? Mind the step and pull up a chair. Look, between you and me, I know I wasn't invited. I'm never exactly welcomed with open arms. I mean, really?

But let's get a few things straight. Who told you life was going to be easy? You can't turn the clock back and I'm here to stay, so you may as well get used to me hanging around, whether you like it or not (harsh but true). Which leads me neatly to my next point.

Sure, I'm pretty nasty. I mess up your body and put your brain in a blender. But I've been kind to you too. Don't laugh - without me, would you really appreciate life so much more than you used to? Would you really make the most of every day? I don't think so. You were quite happily trucking along, making plans, blah blah blah, without a care in the world. Life. Is. Not. That. Simple. See? I helped you change your life, didn't I?

Yes, I know you lost everything, but we'll run through that, shall we? Career? If your employer was going to treat you like that, they weren't worth it anyway. Ditto partner.

He scarpered at the first sign of trouble. I saved you the pain at a future date. And stop worrying about finding someone new. Find yourself first, then think about it. So in a strange kind of way, I simply hastened the process of clearing your life out, didn't I?

And I really do think you should thank me for that. Sure, I prod you and push you over. And? I see you laughing at it now. You turned it round. You used to trip and curse every single time. Now you shrug it off. Life is all about adapting, every single day. Nothing stays the same. And if that's the only thing I can teach you, then I'm happy.

You're doing ok. You faced up to me (and to be frank, you're a teeny bit scary when you do that). I think you are much more powerful than before, despite feeling weaker. Have a think about it. Anyway, I'll leave you with that. And please, no more pity parties. Yawn.

Yours forever,

MS xxx

12th March 2014

A Sad, Wan Little Face

The Teenager has been poorly. To make sure he wasn't blagging, I immediately ran the Playstation Test - waving the controller in front of him to check for a response. Nothing.

Just to make absolutely certain, I resorted to the Nutella Test, offering to fetch him some toast slathered in the stuff. Not a flicker. Oh. It was probably serious.

The Teenager is rarely ill, so when he is, he seems to display a dazzling array of symptoms, as if he's been saving them up for a special occasion. Luckily he made it to the loo in time (and time again), the Bloo was changed and I sloshed a bottle of bleach around (in the toilet, not on The Teenager).

He lay in bed, tossing and turning. I then heard through the rugby-grapevine that a load of kids had been felled by the same bug. All Sunday and into Monday I was the butler/nursemaid. I fetched this, I carried that, I soothed and reassured. I had to work part of Monday so my mum took over, dashing down to my house with sandwiches and treats plus the ubiquitous biscuits for the cat (she's not daft, she hears my mum coming a mile off).

She called me in work - 'Well, he's had half a sandwich, a wee bit of lettuce and some Smarties and the cat's had all her biccies. Oh and I found that dead bird she left outside and put it in your recycling bin, dear. It was a robin, poor thing.'

By Monday evening, he was returning to normal, managing a short Skype call with his friend - 'yeah, it was mega - all over the bathroom, you should have *seen* it.' By Tuesday, he was wolfing down a pie, asked for chocolate and watched a football match on telly. All back to normal. A sigh of relief.

He was packed off to school this morning, totally recovered and no doubt with a stronger immune system but without his chemistry homework completed. All was right with the world again. I got to work. Gah. The boss turns up clutching a medical cupboard full of cough/indigestion/headache/throat tablets. He's unable to eat his usual morning pastry and orders an immune-boosting smoothie at our coffee-house catch up meeting instead of his usual caramel macchiato. Here we go again.

14ᵗʰ March 2014

48 Hours

Ha Lay Loo Ya! Much as I adore The Teenager (and he is totes cute), it's always a little bit lovely to have the house all to myself when he goes to London for the weekend. The house. To myself. For 48 delicious hours. I always have such great plans. This weekend I will mostly:

• Put a face pack and hair mask on.

• Eat a £10 meal deal all on my own (shame I ate the starter and dessert yesterday. Oops).

• Wear a kimono after a long, long shower without being laughed at.

• Talk to the plants, especially Bertie.

• Go to bed early with a pile of magazines and a new book.

• Desperately catch up on Book Club book I have yet to read. We meet on Monday, gah.

• Handwrite a pile of cards to my dear friends I have shamefully neglected recently.

• Listen to music really, really loud on my headphones without worrying that The Teenager is yelling at me from upstairs.

In reality, I will do none of these things. I'm kidding myself. I will mostly be:

- Making inroads into my teetering pile of ironing.

- Organising new house insurance. 'Citing.

- Cleaning the microwave. And maybe the oven if I'm feeling adventurous.

- Changing the cat litter tray.

- Putting clean sheets on the bed.

- Talking to the plants

- Scrubbing the grout in the bathroom with an old toothbrush (strangely therapeutic).

Why do I do this? I should be out, painting the town a slightly murky, dusky pink. I could be theatring, cinemaring, bar hopping, gadding about town. I guess the grass is always greener. When I would like to go out, I can't. When I can't, I'm stunned by inertia (aka laziness).

I will no doubt end up in bed at 7pm, shattered by working all week and being called 'Half Shift' at regular intervals. My cunning plan to learn Japanese over the weekend will be shelved. I will also not be teaching myself macramé. Or decoupage. Or glass painting.

I will stick to one of my first points though. I will blast out 'I Am Woman', shortly followed by 'Those Were The Days My Friend'. And if I'm feeling particularly maudlin,

you can't beat a bit of Velvet Underground. Don't panic.
It's not a pity party. It's a 'can't be bothered' party.

16th February 2014

What Would You Say?

The worst thing about my job is having to listen to commercial radio all day long when I'm on site. Ten songs on a loop, one inane competition, kerrr-aazzy DJ's and endless adverts. But one creepy advert has piqued my interest.

It's by Legal & General, the insurance company. They ask, 'What would you say to your younger self?' i.e. would you tell your 20 year old self to buy life insurance as you will in all likelihood die one day or sign up for critical illness cover as you will probably become very ill at some point? You get the picture.

They trade in fear. Sure, it's great to have fun when you're younger, but It Won't Last and if you're not 'protected', then tough luck. And yes, it's wonderful to find that special person, but hey, they could die. Suddenly. And then where would you be? Tsk.

Anyway, this got me thinking. At the grand old age of (whisper) 40, do I really have anything earth-shattering to say to my younger self? Seems a bit of a pointless exercise, but fun nonetheless. So here goes:

• Never wear stripy tights. And blue eyeshadow doesn't suit you.

- Your heart will be broken but it will mend.

- Childbirth is gobsmackingly painful. Be prepared.

- Experiences are worth far more than material goods.

- It's more fun to have a glass of water in The Dorchester than a glass of champagne down the local.

- Today is the youngest you will ever be, so make the most of it.

- Don't waste money on self-help books. You already have the answers.

- Accept every challenge life throws at you with grace.

I'm feeling every single one of my years right now. The Teenager will be flying the nest within the next couple of years. I have wrinkles. In odd places. I'm a mere ten years away from being eligible for a Saga holiday.

But the whole point of youth is to explore, make mistakes, make more mistakes. Love and lose, fight and fall. It's when we forge our identities. So if I was offered the chance to go back in time, I probably wouldn't take it. All those 'mistakes' taught me valuable lessons.

And would I tell myself I would be diagnosed with MS in my 30's? No way. Why spoil the party?

14th April 2014

I Only Went and Did It

Much excitement chez moi. It seems I'll be working with my friend for the foreseeable future, so I want to try something just for me, and become a … writer. So, I applied for the MA in creative writing and, um, I was offered a place in September. Eeek.

To pay for it, I may need to find a suitably grotty garret and eat marked-down bread every day (baked beans would blow the budget), huddled in moth-ridden blankets - but I feel that will only add to my new persona. In other developments:

> • The Teenager complained his human rights had yet again been violated by my recent refusal to buy him a Domino's pizza and a large bottle of Fanta. You can imagine how *that* conversation went.

> • I have started a 'notebook where I jot down words I don't know the meaning of' in preparation for my course. An expository prologue would denote that this is a Byzantine, Sisyphean task.

> • Strangely, I developed tennis elbow last week without picking up a tennis racket since 1984.

> • I cut my own hair in a moment of frustration. Not to be recommended, although I'm pleasantly surprised at the outcome (after several angsty

days). Plus I'll save a fortune on hair masks, intensive moisturisers, olive oil, eggs, etc...

• The cat continues to bring little field mice into the house and drop them at my feet then bowing and stepping back with an innocent grin before pointing to her food bowl. Must remember to wear socks or slippers in the morning. Mice entrails feel a bit squishy underfoot at 6am.

• The Teenager has lodged an official complaint. I must not, under any circumstances, feed him any of the following: leeks, tomatoes, onions, spring onions, blue cheese of any description, chili flakes, tarragon, mustard, garlic or enchiladas. I have been encouraged to buy food only at shops full of freezers. Anything with chips apparently. And gravy.

Apart from that, life continues as normal. The Teenager is due back in two hours after a long weekend in London. We are off to New York on Wednesday - making good use of my tiny tribunal pay-out. Yup, The Teenager is coming to Manhattan. Watch this space, it should be a blast...

15th April 2014

Ready Or Not

O to the M to the G. We are getting ready for New York. Manhattan. A Times Square hotel. Bonkers. I have two suitcases wide open.

In mine - pyjamas, earplugs, moisturiser, face pack, shower gel, trainers, pen, notebook, clothes (natch), headphones, challenging novel, bubble bath, wet wipes, more wet wipes, NY guide book.... In The Teenager's - shampoo, Lynx, SPACE for all the Tootsie Rolls he plans on buying and selling at school for a premium.

It's weird. I spent a very happy six months living in New York. I was young and daft. A mere 19 years old. And now I'm taking my son there. I lived next door to a Snapples sales-man in the west village. But that was 20 years ago. It's all changed. What will he make of it?

How will I fare with MS and Manhattan? Should I sit in a café and wave The Teenager off? He goes to London every month, so it's not that different? Will he be inspired, as I was? Who knows. But what I do know is his must-do list:

- Tootsie Rolls

- American t-shirts

- A hot dog from a hot dog vendor

- A taxi

- A fire escape

- Steam rising from the metro (underground?)

- McDonalds

- Taco Bell

- Wendy's

24th April 2014

First We'll Take Manhattan

Manhattan. We made it. The Teenager was overwhelmed. The view from our hotel room, the vast array of fast food outlets (natch), the endless shopping for t-shirts, the atmosphere. It was a film set come true.

We sailed around Manhattan, circumnavigated the Statue of Liberty, saw the whole city from the top of the Empire State building, wandered the streets, peered in windows. We chatted to NYPD cops. To Starbucks employees, random people.

For me, New York reignited my love of life. Life and energy were everywhere. I spoke to a mother and daughter from North Carolina, putting in place a bucket wish list. I spoke to Irish bar-tenders who had moved there and lost everything in the storm but were still trucking on, plus he makes the best martinis that side of the Atlantic (The Hyatt, off Times Square).

Anyway, yes, New York was a breath of fresh air. After over two years pretty much house bound through job loss and loneliness, I realised that life goes on. And on. It happens whether I like it or not. I have been a bit of a hermit. So here's what I will take home with me:

- Life is waaaaaay bigger than my little world.

- I can wear what I like, when I like. Even if I am fat (I know, I know).

- There is a whole world out there, ready to explore.

- MS may curtail stuff, but stuff it.

Fair play, MS reared its ugly head. And then some. I was in Macey's and felt the earth move (really). After panicking and looking around me I finally got the picture. It was me. I was on the top floor. But, hey, I had a brand new Ralph Lauren trench coat at 75% off. MS be damned. I went back to the hotel and admired my beautiful coat before conking out for three hours.

19th May 2014

Annual Report

I was handed an opened A4 envelope today by The Teenager, with the words: 's'ok you know, s'not me, s'my teachers, honest, I mean, reallllllly, you know, innit, obvs.'

Yes. School Report Time. First, the good news -he has a 96% attendance record with 0% unauthorised. As for the rest:

- '...he has the potential to be an amazing student...but he procrastinates......'

- '....he is a popular member of the class but can become distracted'

- '...he is a bright pupil but easily distracted....'

- '.....you can do it!'

And so on. So we had The Talk. Of course, his teachers lie. Dreadfully. Tut. Never in my day. I was, and I freely admit it, a girly swot. I was over the moon when I found out he would have the same German teacher as me. At parents' evening a couple of years ago, we had a huge hug (I hadn't seen her since I left for Austria at the age of 18), then she sweetly told me The Teenager would never be reading Brecht in the original. But no matter, he had other talents.

And he does. Many. What's difficult is juggling this hormone-tastic time with general life. Take for example a couple of days ago: Me: Hey, that was a nice dinner, no? Him: Yeah. But I hate MS. Me: Oh. Um. Yeah. Was it the carrots? Him: Hate carrots. Hate MS. Me: And how does that make you feel? (what else should I have said??) Him: Sad.

The next day we had breakfast together in a café. I tentatively raised the subject again - MS, not the carrots. We chatted. We mulled over how both our lives had changed. We shared a latte. MS is horrible.

The Teenager has needed to formulate what has happened to me into words he can understand and pass on and make acceptable for his peer-group, i.e. 'oh, yeah, my mum has MS, just like Jack Osbourne. I know!!!! Wicked (or dench, lush, etc)' The biggest accolade happened the other day: 'I told (friend) all about you and the MS, and he likes you and I like you and he's staying over on Tuesday, so can we have pizza?'

20th May 2014

You Are Now Entering The MS Bubble

Hmmm. It's been pointed out to me that perhaps I live in an MS bubble - I think MS, breathe MS, speak MS. Nothing could be further from the truth.

Fair enough, perhaps I *am* trapped in some kind of bubble, but through no choice of my own. I have always said, if I had a partner, he would be my 'blog'. I could offload, work through feelings, come to resolutions. I don't have that. Therefore, I blog.

• First, I must address the point made by some friends - they know people who don't 'bang on' about having MS. Hmm. I write a blog about MS. (come to my house and we'll chat about anything and everything but not MS - for more than five minutes). Furthermore:

   • My blog is not the whole story. Believe me, you would run for the hills if you heard the whole sorry saga.

   • I have a life outside my blog. Yup!

   •I lost my job thanks to MS and ignorant employers - MS (but I won the tribunal - result!).

   • I nearly flunked Uni - MS.

   • I passed degree and enrolled on an MA - MS.

   • My career path has radically altered - MS.

• My (sadly neglected) dating history has ground to a halt - MS.

So, yes, MS has had an impact on virtually every area of my life. Even down to reading a book. Anything more than 300 pages and it's Kindle, not a paperback. Numb hands are not much fun.

Ditto shampoo bottles. And squeezy ketchup. I was told (by a fellow MSer) that I 'may as well go out with him' as he was 'the best I could hope for now I have MS.' Well, no.

My world has perhaps been shaped and altered by MS, but it in no way defines who I am. I was always go-getting. I was always adventurous. I have always brought up The Teenager to believe that life was out there, ready to be discovered. So, no, MS is definitely not the most important thing in my life. The Teenager is.

22nd May 2014

Happy MS-Versary To Me

On Sunday, it will be two years to the day that I was diagnosed with MS. Two teeny-weeny years, but it feels like a lifetime ago. Unlike my six-month anniversary (totes pretentious sad, no?), this will be a time of positive and uplifting reflection. I am throwing off the black mourning clothes, although I do look rather fetching and dramatic in black. Maybe I'll just keep the wonky black eye-liner. And beret. Anyway, so here I am. Here is my list of things I feel truly grateful for:

- I have moved into the acceptance phase. At Long Last. I've gone from being scared beyond belief, waking in the wee small hours, to being well-informed, if still a little bit scared.

- My relationship with The Teenager is stronger than ever. He went to London one weekend three years ago and came back to a parent who was in hospital unable to speak or walk properly. He was only 11. We've had tears, heart-rending conversations and hugs. Just yesterday he asked me if I was going to die of MS. I was driving at the time, bit awkward, but we chatted about it and I reassured him I would be around long enough to show his great-grandchildren that photo of him sitting naked in a jumbo-sized plant pot when he was two.

• I have a brilliant support network. From our MS team here in Cardiff who are amazing to all you guys I've met through blogging and Twitter.

• I have a fabulous job with my best friend. Ok, so he might snigger when I trip over yet again, or forget what I was saying halfway through a conversation, but he's been great. He employed me as soon as I was sacked from my last job, even though he hates tax-office paperwork with a passion.

• I finally finished my second degree (after much, much wailing and angst) and have signed up for an MA. Never would have happened without MS. It really does make you grasp life with both hands - no pun intended.

This Sunday, as much as I would like to host a tea party or climb some random mountain just to mark the day, I will be in work. Yup. Some things never change *waves to boss*

27th May 2014

What Have I Done?

Well, my MS-versary passed without major incident. I ended a very pleasant evening out still talking fairly intelligently to my friends rather than random trees or street signs (it has been known).

Life was looking good. I was in a good place, feeling, um, good. Until an email pinged on my phone. A weighty document from the university, detailing a reading list, term dates, rules, regulations, how to get a student ID card (yay!) and plagiarism warnings.

Oops.

Have I been a bit too hasty in signing up for an MA? Will my brain have the last laugh? I scanned the book list, the phrases 'developing effective analysis and argument', 'critical thinking skills', 'Harvard referencing' leaping out at me.

Assignments include a 6,000 word novel chapter, a 3,000 short story and a 10,000 word dissertation. Perhaps my expectations have been a little on the low-expectation side. I imagined Creative Writing to be, well, creative and artistic. I had a vision of myself scribbling important thoughts in a battered notebook with a lilac pen.

I would be sitting in a dingy café wearing fingerless gloves and studenty clothes. Me and The Teenager would cook beans on toast and lentil curry on alternate nights, warmed by the glow of our last candle. Perhaps we would visit the market at the end of the day to pick up plums and turnips that had fallen on the floor.

The last time I critically analysed anything, it was a letter from my neurologist detailing the sorry state of my brain, and even then I had to google the long words. This course would be a whole different brain-game. Am I really up to it?

In a bid to calm down, I listened to my 'You Are Intelligent and You Can Do It!' relaxation thingie. Unfortunately this left me more stressed as I couldn't count down my 'Stairway To Success' without losing track of where I was. And when the American voice told me I was a worthy and special being, all I heard was 'you are a special bean'. I snorted with laughter and missed the next bit about creating compartments in my mind where I could store important information. Gah.

In a fit of optimism, I ordered everything from my reading list and I have a new pot of freshly-sharpened pencils on my desk. Am I ready for September? About as ready as I was for my lumbar puncture.

3rd June 2014

Don't Need No Education

The Teenager is sitting some GCSE exams, with the rest to follow next year. I have bought him the Lett's guides, replenished his pen-pot, explained how to write up mind maps and supplied him with a steady stream of juice to refresh his brain. To no avail.

In the middle of cooking dinner yesterday (a home-made curry he refused to eat - tough), the phone rang. 'Mrs Stumbling?' 'Yeeeeees?' 'Well,' and sounding relieved to reach a real, live parent on the phone, regaled me with a tale of woe and lost opportunities. The Teenager could easily reach an A in this subject, but is cruising close to an F, if he's lucky.

The usual - not concentrating, joking around, no proper presentation of coursework. It was a good conversation in some ways. I explained that he has all the support he needs here. Apart from anything else, I've been studying something or other for ten out of his fourteen years. It simply boils down to him being a Teenager who is somewhat lazy. And rude. And...(I could go on and on).

When he came home from school, I summoned him to the kitchen as I was juggling naan bread, a hot grill and a large pot of curry. He saw my face and scarpered, slamming his bedroom door extra loud. He really should have taken GCSE drama. He's quite superb.

I counted the seconds, and sure enough, within 15, loud music was blasting out. The angsty type. I yelled up the stairs - handily, his name has three syllables, so the effect can be quite stern. 'Wha?' 'Come down........NOW.' After a stand-off worthy of a spaghetti western, he sloped into the kitchen, refused dinner (a recent recurring theme), told me his version of events - 'teacher hates me, wasn't doing nuffink wrong, s'not fair.' Stage direction - exit left.

A while later his door opened and his school tie floated downstairs, followed by the door slamming shut again. Not the most rigorous form of protest, but it made me laugh. Which annoyed him.

I can only do so much. Nothing to do with MS. I have just returned from a visit to Staples as his pencil case was stolen and he needs the stuff for exams. He has an exam today. He told me this last night, around 10pm. Stage direction - curtains.

9th June 2014

The Fickle Finger Of Fate

Once upon a time, my career path was set. Then along came the dastardly Evil Bosses who cast me out into the wilderness for daring to bring MS to the boardroom table. Step forward the Good Fairy Goblin Wizard, my best friend, who swiftly put me on his payroll and offered me a job with his construction company, giving me breathing space to find a new one.

One and a half years later, I'm still working with him. I love my job. I adore it. It's flexible, fun and challenging. This friend held my hand all the way through the MS diagnostic process and beyond so probably knows more about MS than I do, thanks to my late-night outpourings of anguish, tears and ridiculous rage against the world.

Sure, when I'm on site (trying to look important and clued up), he sniggers when I trip over a solitary wood-shaving or kick something over for the umpteenth time. He laughs when my bacon buttie suddenly drops from my hand, and he directs me discreetly to a quiet corner when my yawning starts to spread to the labourers.

We've just taken on a huge project, so my job is secure for at least another year, or however long the boss can put up with me (hope he's not reading this). We're tying up loose ends on other jobs before we commit fully to it. Last week, I was with him on a kitchen conversion. My main tasks were to measure up, jot down materials we needed and work out the logistics. Oh, and order a Portaloo for the big job (a very funny conversation with the lovely Emma in Bristol).

We work well together so, without thinking, the boss called out, 'there, no there, yup there, watch your step', and 'pick that blinking cable up before you lassoo your foot in it, you dweeb.'

My work is different every single day. And if I'm having a bad day, I make up for it another time. There's no office politics (a huge positive after the vicious back-stabbing in my last job) no set working times and the men I work with are brilliant. They're old enough to be my sons (eeeeeeeek), so I am a surrogate Agony Aunt/Mother. The Teenager has unwittingly given me plenty of experience.

So, yes, my career has certainly not panned out the way I envisaged. Not even close. That fickle finger of fate. But my job has given me the space to also do what I love most, writing, which is why I signed up for a Masters in creative writing. The best of both worlds. What more could I wish for? p.s. I really do have a pink hardhat.

12th June 2014

A Blessing, Heavily Disguised

Yesterday, I was having a chat with someone I'd never met before. For various reasons, MS popped in to the conversation, as it does. We discussed how it had affected my life, what had changed. Towards the end I said, 'you know what, in some ways, I am blessed.'

Weird word to use. I've thought about this before, but yesterday it really crystalised for me. She seemed perplexed. I tried to explain that a lot of people are well into their 50's/60's or even 70's before a major health crisis appears. To have had this happen in my 30's and to get the chance to totally re-evaluate my life from every perspective is a gift.

MS brought me up short and made me realise just how fleeting and wondrous life can be. I would be most miffed for this to happen at, say 65, and think to myself, 'all those regrets, all those wasted opportunities.' Mind you, I haven't always felt this way, as regular readers will be well aware. The sheer unfairness of it all. The grieving process, the fears, the endless panic.

It didn't help that in my case the MS onslaught was so dramatically sudden - I went to bed one evening and woke up the next morning unable to speak or walk properly.

MS cleared the decks. The uncommitted boyfriend swiftly left the building (see ya! No, I didn't want to marry you either) old family politics diminished in their insignificance and most of my fair-weather friends disappeared in a cloud of, 'honestly, if you need *anything*', whilst stepping/running backwards from the room.

I started to ask what my life was all about. What did it mean? What could I do that would be fulfilling? For me and The Teenager. Which is why I spent my tiny tribunal payout on a trip to New York, the least I could do after all the Teenager had coped with. MS is also the reason I've enrolled on an MA.

And, dear reader, it's the reason I am in touch with a, ahem, personal trainer, to try to instill some body confidence after it's been battered with steroids, meds and far too much comfort food.

I still have fears. I'm still reminded every single day that MS is ever-present. But I think now I am living the life I was meant to live. I'm just hoping the trainer goes easy on me and at least allows me to congratulate myself with a doughnut for picking up the kettle bell, which has been my trusty doorstop for the last two years. We'll see.

18th June 2014

Mirror, Mirror

....on the wall, who's the blobbiest of them all?

Well, me.

MS does the weirdest things to your mind and body. First and foremost, it had the utter cheek to launch an all-out attack on me (itself?). Three years ago, my faithful body drew up the battle lines and hunkered down for a long-term offensive, 'offensive' being the operative word. Bits of me started to go wonky, my mind melted into a goo-like mass and my once-trusted-with-my-life body morphed into a despised stranger. I no longer understood what it was doing, or why.

Then there was the terrifying diagnostic process, which in my case was somewhat helped along by a bountiful supply of comfort food. I didn't care. What was an extra scoop of Mackie's Indulgent Ice Cream between enemies? Or a special offer bag of M&M's? Junk food was a soothing balm to my battered soul.

And finally, the meds, the steroids. Mind you, one of the courses of steroids meant my Christmas tree was put up in record time a couple of years back. And I finally got round to painting anti-mould stuff on the bathroom ceiling. They might taste foul, but boy, the energy!

All this has culminated in my just not recognising myself. Who is this large, scowling person staring back at me from shop windows and inappropriately placed mirrors? (A note to all you zeitgeist-y restaurants and wine bars - mirrors may make your place look bigger, but it's most off-putting when I'm trying to look super-elegant whilst sipping my Martini and carrying on a scintillating conversation, ta).

Anyway, I have reached Crunch(ie) point. I am out of that dark tunnel, blinking into the light of grudging acceptance of this foul illness. And I really don't like what I see. I used to have cheekbones. I still do, with a bit of Sellotape, but I would like my real ones back please. They're buried underneath that chubby face, somewhere.

I would like to banish the bingo-wings. Tone those thighs. Walk tall again, rather than hunching over and scanning the pavements for tripping hazards. To that end, yesterday, I met with my brand, shiny, new personal trainer. And I signed up for a year (sits down, takes a moment).

He's the only person alive who knows my true weight. He is inspiring and understanding and won't put me through gym-bunny crazy intensive workouts.

He's got a lovely holistic approach, perfect for a systemic illness like MS which affects pretty much every single part of your life. As I write, I have the polish ready to clean up my doorstop kettlebell. I've ordered a dri-fit pair of leggings and t-shirt. I am petrified.

29ᵗʰ June 2014

Eyes Wide Open

I have developed an annoying symptom recently. Some evenings, when I'm reading a book or watching an exciting TV programme (Hannibal, Pretty Wicked Moms), I go from wide awake to instantly zonked. No reprieve.

It starts right out of the blue; my eyes start rolling and I'm pinned to the sofa, completely aware of what's coming next - total oblivion. In that slim interim, I know I should get up and walk around, problem is I just can't. Its suddenness is frightening.

Apart from that, The Teenager sneaks downstairs and slurps down countless yoghurts while I'm in the Land of Nod. He probably also clones my credit card to buy online games, who knows?

Anyway, I had my review with the neurologist (a very nice man - *waves*) just over a week ago. When he asked me if I had anything I was concerned about, I launched into the saga of my numb big toe, my odd left foot, my odd right foot and this most peculiar Insta-Sleep (just add yawns).

He prescribed me Amantadine, warning me to take them no later than 2pm, otherwise I would be up all night - I wish. Yes, I was sorely tempted. But, I took them as instructed and nothing happened for almost a week. Then, blam, I was......awake. Fully.

The grass was green and the bluebirds were singing. My life was suddenly in blinding Technicolor. I worry though that the tablets mask the underlying symptoms. Am I pushing myself too far? Will I reach a point of collapse? Will this new-found energy enable me to exercise more?

Bearing in mind that last Monday, the few squats I attempted with my lovely trainer led to four days of agony. I'm not joking. I walked up and downstairs at home like a crab, meh. Also, the tablets have given me the most amazing dreams, so vivid that when I wake up in the morning I have to remind myself what is real and what is imaginary. I have the most wonderful conversations with friends and family, but I find out to my dismay that they are entirely one-sided.

I will keep trying with the tablets. I made the mistake of telling my boss. He offered to trade me two packets of Jaffa Cakes for a tablet. I wasn't tempted. Much.

6th July 2014

Adventures in Blunderland

I am about to start the third week of my New Me regime, i.e. ELF (Eat Less, Fatty). My lovely trainer has shown me some exercises to boot my metabolism out of its lengthy hibernation, and amazingly, it appears to be working.

Combined with snacking on Brazil nuts and sunflower seeds rather than Cheez-E-Puffs or Curly Wurlys, I am feeling a tad virtuous. It hasn't all been plain sailing though. I bought one of those resistance band thingies, with two (pink) handles. The trainer showed me some smart moves I could do at home. Easy, no?

The plan was to sling the band round the pillar in my living room and use that as resistance, pulling away to tackle my burgeoning bingo-wings. 15 reps, rest, 15 reps, rest, 15 reps, rest. Who said exercise was hard work? This would be a doddle. I could watch telly from the pillar, catching up with my favourite junk programmes, i.e. 'I Wanna Marry Harry'. Fabulous time management and I duly gave myself a pat on the back.

First problem, pillar is actually quite large, so I ended up hugging the darned thing to wrap the band round it, just as The Teenager came downstairs, rolled his eyes and, seeing me incapacitated, made a break for the fridge.

Right. handles sorted, move forward a bit and....I was off. Did my reps, felt a little bit of a 'burn', rested, started again. Meh. Adverts. I always fast forward, so I reached for the controller, trying to put both handles in one hand. Almost there......thwack. Couldn't do it, the resistance band thingie flew backwards, one handle whacking me smack in the eye. The Teenager rolled his eyes and darted back upstairs.

I kicked the stupid band thingie around the floor a few times (it's still exercise) and decided to try on my new sports bra instead. Well. Whoever invented this torture device deserves to be pelted with soggy rugby socks. I ended up with one arm stuck in the air and the other attached to my thigh. After struggling to free myself from the evil contraption for over five minutes (and bouncing over to the window to close the curtains), I flopped onto my bed, limp, weak and exhausted.

I will not be beaten. The ELF Challenge continues..

13th July 2014

Not Dressed Up, Nowhere To Go

Something disturbing happened the other day. I was out with a friend, dressed casually, sipping a glass of wine with two hands in one of those faux-bonhomie wine bars with 'ironic' artwork and staff with obligatory piercings/sullen expressions/selective deafness. But I digress.

Two couples entered, both women in spray-on dresses, dazzling white teeth, teetering heels and big, big hair. After looking longingly at their heels (sigh), I clocked that their partners were much younger. Nothing wrong with that. After collecting their drinks from the bar, they perched on the chairs next to us, so I couldn't help but do a nosy.

The men (boys) seemed unable to sit still without squeezing the women every five minutes, in, ahem, not-totally-appropriate places. I'm no prude but this was seriously interrupting my fascinating conversation about my new Gorgonzola and steak recipe and I quickly lost my thread.

So we bar-hopped to the next place. Five minutes later, the same couples came tumbling through the door. To cut a long story short, I found myself in a place surrounded by eerily similar-looking twosomes, like some kind of weird parallel zone. 'Yell at me if I ever get like that just to get a man when I'm that old' I remarked smugly, casting my beady eye around the mayhem.

My former friend choked on his drink and said 'they're our age, look, that one's got a 'Still Flirty At 40' badge on and that one's definitely had Botox. They're all in their 40's. Like us.' He was right. I sulked the rest of the evening, lying awake later that night pondering my Sad Single Situation.

Is this the only way to date in my 40's? As if it wasn't hard enough being divorced with a grumpy Teenager, a rude cat and to top it all, MS, does entering my fifth decade condemn me to a life of body-con crash diets, hair extensions and laughing politely when my date burps the Welsh national anthem?

The only alternative seems to be joining an evening class in the autumn, perhaps signing up to Very Hot Indian Cooking, in the hope that I will find my soulmate over some poppadoms and mango chutney.

I reckon the powers that be in adult education should start a brand-new class for 'peeps who want to meet other peeps but have to pretend to be interested in Very Hot Indian Cooking or Yoga for Complete and Utter Numpties'. Heels and hair extensions preferred, but not essential.

22nd July 2014

No (Sigh), I'm Not Drunk

Vertigo. Vile, evil vertigo: 'a sensation of whirling and loss of balance' according to my dictionary.

There's two reasons you'll get no sympathy for sharing this MS symptom with anyone else. First, if you say, 'ooh, me vertigo's playing up something awful today' as you fumble blindly for something to hold on to, you'll inevitably hear, 'oh yeah, I hate heights too.' (Grrr). Or they'll say, 'ha! Thought it was wine o' clock and you'd already started on the Mother's Ruin' followed by them imitating your rolling gait in a totally exaggerated fashion.

This happened to me a couple of days ago and my 'audience' was none other than The Teenager, so I kind of expected just a tiny bit of compassion on his part. Not a bit of it. I was helping him pack his bag for London, i.e. I was holding up clothes for his Romanesque thumbs up or down. (Looks up from his phone for a nanosecond - snort, snigger) 'Muuuuuuum, I know I'm going away for a week but did you have to start the celebrations early? Like, really?' (imitates my rolling gait).

I did my best to explain in a non-worrying manner, playing it down, good parent that I am, trying to move ever so slowly so I didn't fall flat on my face. 'Vertigo? Yeah, I get that too. Dad took me up The Gherkin in London and I was like, woah, bit scary. But I didn't look like you do. And I got some sick (sic) photos.'

After waving my little cherub off to the bus-stop I sank onto the sofa. The world stopped moving for a while, if I closed my eyes. But then I felt sick. My phone went. 'Muuuuuuuum. You know when I get back next week, seeing as you'll have missed me, can I have a Domino's? Pleeeeeeeaaaaaase?'

'Sweetheart, you've been gone all of three minutes. We'll talk about it later.' 'Meanie.'

The rest of my first evening of child-freeness was spent attempting to walk the length of my house without veering off to one side. The world didn't stop moving. Everything was spinning faster than I could walk. I gave up and went to bed early, mega early.

The next morning, I woke up to a panicked message from a friend, saying she couldn't get hold of me last night and was worried. I explained I'd gone to bed with vertigo at 8-ish and had put my phone on silent. 'Oh yeah, I hate heights too. What were you doing? Rock climbing?'

29th July 2014

Is It Time For An Update?

Just out of interest and because I've been bored in work recently (sorry, boss), I've been asking people what MS conjures up in their minds. My random and unscientific survey threw up some depressing results; according to my motley panel of vox-poppers, MS is:

• An older person's illness

• An illness that means you have to give up work as soon as you're diagnosed

• An illness with no treatment

• An illness that will propel you into a wheelchair soon after diagnosis

• An illness that absolutely everyone has a story about, normally, 'oh my auntie/great-grandad/batty neighbour had that, dreadful it was. How they suffered' (sad face)

It seems MS has a serious image problem.

When I tell them MS is the most common neurological illness in young people and is generally diagnosed between the ages of 20 and 40, they're astounded and/or disbelieving. So what's going on? Is it that we've made astonishing progress over the last 30 years, but the image remains the same?

Take my dad, for example. He was diagnosed at the age of 28 and died at 35 in 1978 from complications arising from his MS. There was no treatment and he was sent home with a walking stick and back then, MS was even referred to as 'creeping paralysis'.

Five years later, in 1983, the MS Society gave a £1 million research grant for the purchase of the first MRI scanner in the world to be solely dedicated to MS research, changing the way MS is diagnosed. A decade later, in 1993, the first three MS specialist nursing posts were created.

Today, there are 270 MS nurses in the UK. There are currently 10 licensed disease modifying drugs and 8 more are in the pipeline. Is it simply that MS is mostly an 'invisible' illness, only making itself apparent to everyone else at its more serious stages?

What is the true picture of MS? Is it time to re-brand MS?

· 1st August 2014

Just Gimme The Cake (And No-One Gets Hurt)

It's almost that time of the year again - whisper - hint - one more candle? Yup, even before I've recovered from my 40th birthday (or to put it more starkly, the first year of my fifth decade), my 41st rolls round in less than two weeks.

I'm at the very great age now that people start putting fewer candles on my cake, not more, i.e. four rather than forty. Perhaps making up the deficit with an indoor sparkler. Fire hazard? Sparing my feelings? Or just cheapskates?

And not only that, my cute, bonny wee baby turns FIFTEEN a mere week later, the effrontery. He was actually due before my birthday in 1999, but was so lazy he decided to doze off and hang around a bit longer.

Anyway, with the onset of August, and the inevitable countdown to Christmas (grrr), it's time for me to gaze at my naval once more. I do a lot of that. It doesn't get me very far, but at least I'm seen to be trying.

So what do I wish for this birthday? Looking back at all those fruitless wishes of yesteryear (My Little Pony with the lightning strike, Cabbage Patch Doll twins, Fuzzy Felts At The Zoo) I won't be getting my hopes up. There are a few reasons for this:

- I pretty much have all I could possibly want. My joy was complete when I brought my new bread-maker home a few days ago. And my new set of ceramic pans arrived this afternoon. Bliss.

- I am grateful for all I have. Even when I hold my breath on entering The Teenager's Lair. I've just been up to check - four plates, three forks (should I be worried?), a pyramid of coke cans on his windowsill, a pile of GCSE revision books stuffed into the corner and a pair of swimming trunks on the floor.

- I have to save all my angst and energy for September, when I start my MA. I am now fully enrolled and fully scaring myself silly.

- After it threw that curve-ball of vertigo at me a few weeks ago, MS seems to be on half-days for the summer. It won't last, but I can pretend.

- It's raining. Goodbye hot weather, heeeeelllllllooooooo cool breezes and rain. Lots of it. Uhthoff's, begone.

Before The Official Date, I am chillaxing (ooh, get me), in the knowledge that this month will be Cake Month. Oh, and the next. It'll be my two year Blogging Anniversary. How did that happen?

18th August 2014

Older. Not Wiser

I clung on as long as I possibly could. On my birthday last week, I loudly proclaimed that, actually, *actually*, I wasn't technically 41 until 8.04pm, so basked in the fading glow of my 40th year for most of the day.

I had a leisurely morning, a leisurely lunch with my mum and a leisurely evening with a friend. Very leisurely. Anyway, after blowing out my candle (singular - I'm now too old to merit one per year) and making a desperate wish (nope, not telling), I scribbled a list of everything I would achieve over the next twelve months, now I was of a Grand Old Age:

- I will create a Capsule Wardrobe. A classic trench-coat, several well-cut pairs of trousers and a few silk blouses that hang 'just so'. Plus some select pieces of discreet, yet classy jewellery and a couple of well-chosen scarves, which I will learn how to tie in many different ways, like all the French woman do.

- Likewise, I will ditch the student wardrobe I've been cultivating for the last few decades. I will consign my 'It's Your Round' t-shirt to the charity shop pile, along with my Gap hoodie, washed so many times it's faded from bright green to vomity-puce.

- I will begin a proper skincare regime, with different creams for different parts and different times of the day. Day cream, night cream, afternoon cream, eye cream, neck cream, ear cream and hand cream. I will be slathered.

- I will consider a National Trust membership, which will give me unlimited access to three thousand sites, ensuring a delightful day out every weekend for the next two hundred years. I will not go straight to the gift shop/ye olde café; I will instead join a guided tour and follow the held-aloft umbrella with all the other tourists. However, I will still buy a jar of honey/jam from the gift shop before leaving.

- I will learn how to cook and love risotto. And a proper Sunday lunch, rather than going for a Carvery, along with a twenty-deep queue of other people. Who nick all the roasties before my turn. And steal all the gravy, tsk.

- I will no longer hide the fact I highlight TV programmes I want to watch in the Radio Times, with my special fluorescent pen.

- I may invest in a foot-spa. And one of those things that makes your bath ripple like a jacuzzi.

Yup, I have a plan. I already feel older than my years with this pesky MS - the cog fog, the pavement-watching, the dozing off in front of the telly. Should I embrace it?

Thinking about it, maybe I shouldn't. I've just had a letter from the university I'll be joining in September. A lovely invitation to Fresher's Week. Really. Should I stay or should I go?

20th August 2014

The Secret Diary of Stumbling, Age 37 and ¾

I flicked through my MS diary the other day. Looking back over the heavily-scribbled (and, yes, tear/coffee/wine-stained) pages, it charts my confusion, fear and ignominious entry into a whole new world, complete with a seemingly impenetrable language all of its own.

Trusted health websites always advise you to document everything, from the very first inkling that something is wrong - comes in handy for meeting with a Consultant who may just allocate you seven minutes (including an awkward silence when fumbling taking shoes off - will he notice my holey, mismatched socks?), if you're lucky.

And they may bark random, medically-sounding words at you. So I did. A bit like swotting up for appearing on Mastermind, with specialist-subject questions fired every 18 seconds. I failed. Miserably. I was sent home with a leaflet about MS fatigue and the MS relapse telephone number. But I didn't have MS? Confused? Me too. I didn't understand the 'multiple' in multiple sclerosis. D'oh.

One of my first entries, back in June 2011 is, 'why am I so hot?? Mum thinks it could be an early menopause, grrrrr. Nooooooooooo!!!' Ha! Looking back, that would have been the least of my worries, Tena Lady adventures to one side. And anyhow, I was quite enjoying the flushed-milkmaid visage I seemed to be rocking, after years of hovering just above the 'palest of the pale Celtic face look', i.e. close to corpse-like. Or Twilight.

Quite suddenly though, the language gets more technical- I have oligoclonal bands in my CSF, I have lesions in the subcortical, periventricular and deep white matter suggestive of demyelination. I am diagnosed with CIS. Nope, no idea.

According to my diary, I called the MS nurse later that month to ask about the MS hug, an excruciating tightening around my ribs. Normal. What about not being able to write properly? Normal. Pins and needles? Normal. Foot drop. Yup, you've guessed it. Over the next few months, I moved from CIS to possible to probable MS, as if I were on an evil, unstoppable conveyor belt.

I called the MS nurse again. Electric shocks in my neck? Normal. Falling over? Normal. Slurred speech? Normal. Stabbing pains? Normal. Wouldn't it be great to have a pain that wasn't connected to MS?

May 2012. My last relapse (until February 2014). My hands. Of all things. Crockery was smashed left, right and centre, my mum bought me plastic tumblers and my friends had enormous fun cheering me as I dropped things without warning. And all along, the excruciating, tedious, soul-destroying fatigue.

Late May 2012. Diagnosed. At last. An absolute dichotomy. Utter relief mixed with utter terror. The diary's closed now. I keep my new notes elsewhere. Thanks to cog-fog though, I haven't a clue where they are.

27th August 2014

My Double Life

I live in two very real worlds, and it's becoming increasingly harder to tell which is which. I started taking Amantadine a few months ago in a final, desperate attempt to combat crippling fatigue. You know the type; not the 'ooh, d'you know, I quite fancy a ten-minute shut-eye', but the 'must. lie. down. now. or. else. the. cat. gets. it.'

After a few weeks of, 'hmmm, is it working or is it me hoping it's working?' Blam. I was quite suddenly...awake. Which was novel and lovely. I sailed right past the witching hour of 11am, sped past the goblin hour of 1pm and sauntered in a desultory fashion through the demonic hour of 4pm. I was owning this tiredness malarky.

Until, one weird morning. I woke, upset after having had an argument with a good friend the previous evening. Keen to build bridges, I called them; 'Hey, s'me! Soooo sorry about yesterday! I honestly do like what you've done with the bathroom, really I do.'

'Huh?'

'You know, what we were talking about? When I laughed at your tiles? Didn't mean to, honestly, chocolate brown with green lotus-thingies is gorgeous. Let me make it up to you. Brunch?'

'Huh? And what's wrong with the tiles? You on something?'

Oh. Turns out, I didn't speak to them the evening before at all. I dreamt the whole thing. Not just in Technicolour, but with Panavision, 3-D, total recall Dream-Vision. I could swear it happened. But it didn't.

I forumed it. Ah. Two strange side effects of Amantadine - lack of appetite (not strange, added bonus, surely?) and vivid, disturbing dreams/nightmares.

Since then, I've been ummming and ahhhing. It's incredible to be wide awake. However, I do now struggle to get up in the morning, not a problem I've ever had before. I feel drugged. Which I guess I am. I'm weighing up the pros and cons and am still not sure which way to go. I've heard from a lot of people who've been driven to abandon the medicine due to the nightmares/parallel universe reality. I'm going to give it a few more months.

Last night, I had a wonderful conversation with The Teenager. We put the world to rights and before he left the room (after a great big bear-hug), he put out the rubbish bags, promised to tidy the bathroom and fed the cat. Yeah, I know. As if?

2nd September 2014

Dim? Some

I was with the boss one morning last week; we were
driving to a warehouse to buy something or other for our
latest project. He pointed towards the humungous Tesco
Extra on our left, saying, 'it's been refurbished, there's a
Costa there now too.' 'Oh, um, great! Must check it out,
but you know my heart lies with Ocado.'

We got the something or other from the warehouse,
loaded the van up and drove away. 'Hey, boss! Did'ya
know that Tesco's has had some kind of makeover.
Someone told me. And Costa's has opened. That one, over
there.' Silence.

Then, 'are you winding me up?' 'Nope, boss. Just know
you love your Costa coffee with the caramel swirly thing.'
'Yeeeeeees (very, very, slowly), but ten minutes ago I told
you about it. You're freaking me out.'

'Oh.' 'Your memory, honestly' - then all I heard was
the word 'dim'. 'Oi! I'm not dim. I won a medal once. For
badminton.'

'Nooooooooooooo (very, very, slowly), I said you're like
a dimmer switch. Sometimes very bright but other times,
you know, dimmer. More dim. No, not dim. Just not as
bright. But not dim as such. You know what I mean.'
sulks all the way to the meeting with the architect

But, he had a point. My memory over the last six weeks has been atrocious. Embarrassingly so. I asked my mum, 'I know I'm ancient now, but was your memory this bad when you were 41?' Mums are a polite bunch, aren't they? 'Well, dear, we're all different. We all have strengths and weaknesses. We all find our unique place in the world. But yes, your memory is dire.'

The Teenager plays on this - 'But you said, you *said* I could have a Dominos. Is your memory playing up again? Don't forget you said we could get a dog. AND, remember that £20 I owe you? I'm so happy I paid you back' (he didn't. I know this for a fact). Nice try.

Anyway, on the one hand, it's a great cop-out (pesky MS cog fog), but on the other, I am liable to be hoodwinked on a regular basis, plus I just can't remember anything important. I have to write everything down, to the point that when I walk through my house, I'm accosted by a forest of post-it notes. Which I can't remember writing. What does 'T-hhhhhhh!! CJ R' even mean?

And as for Costa Coffee. I haven't been yet. Did I tell you they opened one in my local Tesco Extra?

21st September 2014

Wot I Did On My Holidays

...or rather, wot I didn't do. Every summer, I scribble down a long list of all the mind-expanding cultural and educational activities I will partake in. Amongst others, I will endeavour to:

> • sign up for a three-day pottery course, throwing (literally) eclectic pots and wonky vases

> • pack a posh picnic, cunningly cultivated from the best of Lidl, and recline elegantly on the grass in the park, listening to live music

> • leave my hair unwashed for a week and watch the sunrise at Stonehenge on the longest day of the year

> • ~~endure~~ watch lots of subtitled films at the local arts cinema and be able to take part in the ~~pretentious~~ lively discussion afterwards

> • visit a food fair and pay triple for a lump of grotty cheese, but feel rather virtuous at the same time

You get the idea. That list is now in the bin. The closest I got to anything cultural was to buy one of those jumbo-CD packs of classical music from the local charity shop to listen to in the car, realising too late that one disc would stick forever on Chopin's piano concerto No. 2 in F minor, 2nd movement.

Instead, I worked a lot. Despite numerous pleas to the Teenager such as, 'C'mon, come on a day trip with your old mum, we'll have fun! We'll pack a Thermos and buy a tin of pear drops', he refused to budge, preferring instead to play football with his friends every day, even though he's in a rugby team. Kids.

For my birthday, The Teenager bought me an iTunes card and slowly, very slowly, explained how to redeem it. He recommended several memory apps and another one that pings when it's time to take your medicine. In return, I stopped his pocket money.

The highlight though, must be GCSE results day, which happened to fall on The Teenager's birthday. I plied him with an All-You-Can-Eat-And-Then-Some-Breakfast buffet at the Toby Inn (only £3.99, but mushrooms - bizarrely - is there a shortage? - and drinks are extra).

Anyway, he refused to pick up his results, as he didn't want to ruin his birthday. I drove past his school twelve times, pointing out all the happy kids clutching bits of paper, driving swiftly past the crying girls on their mobiles, but still, nope. He wouldn't go.

So I did what any good parent would do and collected them myself. Bit embarrassing. Had to show ID, sign a form, swear allegiance to the examining board and explain in less than 100 words why The Teenager wasn't there himself. I passed. And, brilliantly, so did The Teenager. Highest marks possible.

I drove back home and opened the door to The Teenager pacing the room, biting what was left of his nails. I put on my best sad face, wiped a tear away and gave him The Look. 'Hah! Gotcha. You're a star!' Stunned silence, then he ran towards me for a huge hug before launching into a whirlwind of social media.

And that, in a nutshell, was my summer. Fleeting but, um, memorable. Next year, I'm taking a caravan in Tenby.

7th October 2014

Drowning, Not Waving

Oh dearie, dearie me. Oh my. I started the Masters course in Creative Writing last week. How hard could it possibly be? I love reading. I love writing. Simple?

Er, no. I am a fish out of water. Or prawn. It started so well. I made my way to induction, swimming and elbowing against the tide of children headed for the canteen. They were very, very young and I felt very, very old. Mumsy. Grey.

Got my ID card. The woman who took my photo said, 'you can smile you know love, it's not Crimewatch.' I grimaced, picked up my card and joined the young folk in the classroom. And I loved it - learning something new. Filled with enthusiasm, the first lecture loomed. Wasn't too bad, took notes, swotted up.

Then a different lecture about research methods. Without warning, the tutor switched to Swahili and the four hours passed in a blur of 'why am I here, what am I doing and when will they unmask me and chuck me out?'

Then, the first writing assignment. I knew I could do this. I've been writing a form of flash fiction for two years with this blog, each post around 400 words but (hopefully) conveying so much more. I was chuffed with my effort, slaved over it, rewrote it, obsessed about it.

Let's just say, I Don't Get It. I am panicking. I wrote a terrible story. I adore my course, I love the research. I just don't think I have what it takes.

17th October 2014

Boing Boing

An abundance of energy is an elusive pipe dream for someone with MS. A month or so ago, I would have traded my cat's soul for just a pinch of the wonder stuff (sorry, Dora).

I should be more careful what I wish for. My thyroid has decided to go bonkers, a result of the Alemtuzumab treatment and I am bouncing off the walls like a super-charged bouncy ball. I'm averaging around 4 hours of sleep a night, and most of that is disturbed, as I lie there counting the spiders on the ceiling.

However, always one to look on the bright side, I am squealing with unadulterated pleasure at being able to fit into my skinny jeans, once relegated to a dark cupboard, stained with tears. The weight loss is nothing short of a miracle and before I start the thyroid medicine, I am savouring every moment.

I can't pass a mirror or shiny surface without pausing and turning this way and that, buzzing with delight. I have lost my appetite. No, really! I pass on the doughnuts, the Wotsits and even my beloved bacon butties and instead nibble on toast or Brazil nuts.

Another upside is stamina when it comes to the Masters. My third attempt at flash fiction was fabulous (IMHO). The words flowed, no editing necessary. At 3am

I emailed it over to my tutor, sat back with a sigh and caught up with Jerry Springer.

I am speeding through my research books for my first essay, post-it notes flying, fluorescent pen whizzing along the pages. I am a demon. I can't keep up with myself. The house is sparkling and my cordless vacuum is on constant recharge, just like me. I concoct marvellous meals, ready for The Teenager to diss and put to one side before he whips out a Domino's menu and a sad face.

I can't keep still, my legs tremble and jig endlessly. I bump in to walls, trip down the stairs and am nurturing an impressive collection of bruises. It won't last. It can't. I am burning out, ready for the inevitable crash. I am scared of going back to the bad old days when I sleep in the afternoon and nod off during Downton Abbey.

I go back to the doctor on Tuesday when she will put a stop to my fun with meds. The clock starts now and in no time at all, I will be waiting for the sad ping of ready meals and ignoring the dust. Until then, I will handcraft some candles for Christmas presents, paint the walls and clean the taps with a toothpick.

And dust the lampshades, organise my food cupboards, carve a pumpkin, re-pot my plants......before it's too late.

23rd October 2014

Goodbye, Dear Meds

Goodbye, Amantadine. Goodbye to the zipping energy you once gave me. I will miss you. Goodbye to all that. My house will lapse into slovenly-ness again. I will become a stranger to my pink duster, my Febreze and my Vanish stain-remover.

My new thyroid medicine is crossing over with it, making me sleep in every morning then rendering me Bonkers-Stupid with energy five minutes later. I am on a crazy rollercoaster in the twilight world between medicines.

I don't watch telly anymore; the unfolding drama behind my eyes more than makes up for it. As the new meds could suppress my immune system, I have made up some rules for The Teenager:

- You must take your shoes off (including rugby boots) at the door, rather than leaving them on the stairs so I can trip over them.

- Pizza is dangerous.

- You have to wash your hands immediately upon entering the house.

- Pizza could carry nasty bits.

- We shouldn't share towels, so stop nicking mine.

- Pizza is lethal and Dominoes has gone bust.

So, on the one hand, I have a bizarre amount of energy, until the thyroid meds do their bit, but on the other, I am withdrawing from Amantadine, which used to lift me up into stratospheric delights. I am up, then down.

Like yesterday. I had a lecture that evening and was on a medicine-induced high all day, until I sat down and took out my notes. Which had mysteriously disappeared. I was jolted from my torpor by the tutor calling my name and I mumbled an incoherent reply.

I jotted down some squiggles and tried to look present and correct, which was pretty difficult, as I leaned over every time he looked away from me, inching ever closer towards the floor. I was supposed to be back at work today, but woke three minutes before the boss was due to pick me up. I called him in a panic. 'muh, s'wake, s'am'.

He told me he had got me a coffee and would drop it in before driving TO WORK. He did so with a dramatic sigh, handing it to me with a tut and I'm sure I heard him mumble 'easy life' under his breath.

Things will return to normal. I will yawn before midday. I will eat bacon butties again. In the medical meantime, I will zip around, eyes staring and parents will shuffle their children away from me.... luckily it's Hallowe'en soon.

24th October 2014

It's A Hard Life, Being a Student

It truly is.   Especially the evening lectures, when The Teenager cranks up the guilt:

'Can you bring me back some sweets?'

'Nope, there's carrot sticks in the fridge.'

'Can you bring me back a drink?'

'Nope, there's Council Pop in the tap.'

'I need help with my homework.'

'Welsh isn't one of my languages.'

And with that, he strops off upstairs and turns his music up.

When I get back later, he's slumped on the sofa chucking the carrot sticks at re-runs of Countdown. Anyway, apart from that, it's the essays that are my main challenge right now. I had imagined, when signing up for a Masters in Creative Writing, I would be stumbling around in artistically-put-together clothes (garments?), staring at the clouds then scribbling long words and my meaningful impressions of life in a shiny new notebook.

There were two problems with this. First, MS brain has reduced my observations to, 'the clouds were pink. And white. And a little bit fluffy'. And, 'the cat ran away.

And then came back.' Second, I hadn't expected to write essays about writing essays. I had no idea there were so many theories and '-isms' in writing.

I am currently staring at a stack of books about ethnography as a research method. Out of the eight books, I have found five quotes, and two of them say pretty much the same thing.

The university library is a scary place, full of very young intelligent-looking people. And it's very, very quiet. They can hear me scanning and dropping my piles of books a mile away. The machine hates me and the librarians at the desk glare at me.

I also have to write a portfolio of short stories by the end of December. This is going ok, but I seem to be writing very dark stuff. Ho hum. No idea why. But, as with everything over the last three years, I am nothing if not determined. My putty brain is being stretched to capacity.

And I have decided to, gulp, publish the last two years of my blog as a book. At least I can then call myself a writer/author/deluded. I think.

I told The Teenager about my grand literary plans and he stared at me aghast. However, he quickly recovered and suggested ideas for new blog posts I could write about him. I interrupted him and told him the blog wasn't fiction. He muttered something under his breath in Welsh, swiped the last scone and disappeared.

5th November 2014

MS Is What You Make It

A while back, I never thought I'd write this post.

MS was an ugly intruder, returning again and again, chipping away at everything I once held as true. It took my health, of course. But it took more than that.

It spirited away my social life (who wants a friend who trips over when sober? And cries down the phone?). It stole my son's transition into teenagerhood - it was marred by worry and fear. It stole my career.

In essence, it took my future. And it tried to take the very core of me, my spirit.

Well, MS, be damned. You can get away with the trembling, the nerve pain, the stumbling. But I will still barricade the gates so you won't destroy me entirely.

I've been to hell and back and have still not fully recovered. I live in fear of the treatment not working and I've already had a relapse, plus complications (I admit, the over-active thyroid has short-term delights, such as my miraculous weight loss, but it won't last and the Wotsits are already calling...).

My hands don't work properly and the foot drop is verging on the comical, which my bruises bear witness to. I am covered in them.

MS is horrendous. It sneaks up and unleashes a bewildering array of symptoms on us. But if you can come to terms with the fact that Life Will Never Be The Same, you're already halfway there (honestly).

Your families may ignore you and you will probably lose friends. You may also lose your job, as I did (don't forget, I won the legal case). But. For all that, you will transition into a whole new way of living. You will adapt and you will overcome, to coin a tired phrase. Some of you are happy to say that you have MS, MS doesn't have you. Well, it does. But! The way you receive and react to that news is the key to living a brighter future. .

We cannot deny it's a nasty existence. It is right here, right now and it always will be. So we adjust to new ways of living, despite this foul illness.

We can do this, right?

ABOUT THE AUTHOR

Barbara was born in Glasgow way back in the 1970's and moved to South Wales when she was 14.

She has lived and worked in Austria, Scandinavia, New York and Hawaii in jobs as varied as au-pair, translator, homoeopath and clinic receptionist.

Barbara was diagnosed with multiple sclerosis (MS) in 2012 and was subsequently unfairly dismissed from her job. She started blogging about life with MS the same year at www.stumblinginflats.com; the blog is now read in over 100 countries.

She is currently working for a friend's company and is studying for an MA in Creative Writing. She still has no idea what she wants to do when she grows up.

When not hanging around doctor's waiting rooms or having blood tests, she enjoys attempting to perfect the anguished-writer persona in cafés where she scribbles nonsense in her notepad and ponders life.

She lives in Cardiff with her son, The Teenager and a cat.

CONTACT ME

If you want to read more, head over to www.stumblinginflats.com. I'm still blogging random thoughts about life with MS and would love to hear from you.

You can email me at barbarastensland@hotmail.com or contact me through Twitter: @MS_Stumbling.

Printed in Great Britain
by Amazon